Progress in
Cancer Treatment
by Orthomolecular, Food, and Water Medicine

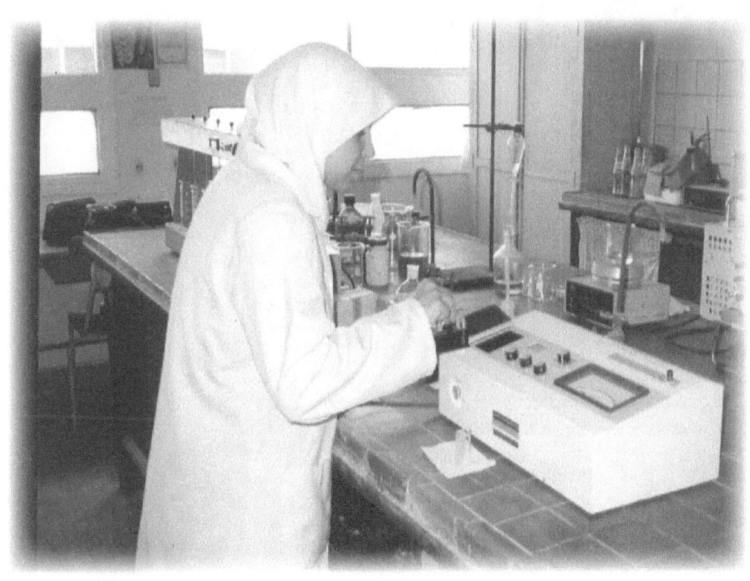

Dr. Badawi and Dr. Khowdiary

Order this book online at www.trafford.com
or email orders@trafford.com

Most Trafford titles are also available at major online book retailers.

Printed in the United States of America.

ISBN: 978-1-4669-8536-0 (sc)
ISBN: 978-1-4669-8538-4 (hc)
ISBN: 978-1-4669-8537-7 (e)

Library of Congress Control Number: 2013904599

Trafford rev. 03/11/2013

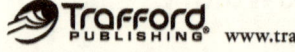 www.trafford.com

North America & international
toll-free: 1 888 232 4444 (USA & Canada)
phone: 250 383 6864 ♦ fax: 812 355 4082

Subject Index

Acknowledgment

With my great appreciation to *my* Ph.D. research student, *Prof. Dr. Amal Abdel Hafeez.* She was the first appreciation rate graduate at the College of Girls—Ain Shams University and then progressed till she became professor of applied chemistry at my department in Egyptian Petroleum Research Institute. She was the Good and Creative Innovation Example, who indefatigably participated in countless scientific research works.

Dr. Abdelfattah M. Badawi
Professor, Applied Surfactant Laboratory
Egyptian Petroleum Research Institute, Nasr City, Cairo, Egypt
(General Secretary for the International Society of Therapeutic, Experimental, and Clinical Research [Bastia, France])

I introduce acknowledgment for *Prof. Dr. Amal* for her support, guidance, and helpful advice throughout my work. Late *Prof. Amal* was a cancer victim and departed from our world on the seventh of October 2010.

Dr. Manal M. Khowdiary
Associate Professor, Applied Surfactant Laboratory
Egyptian Petroleum Research Institute, Nasr City, Cairo, Egypt

Preface

A study was conducted by Dr. Haddad, professor of oncology and nuclear medicine therapy, Faculty of Medicine, Cairo University, and revealed increased level of carcinogenic diseases in Egypt during the past two decades to reach a fourfold rate over the previously recorded rate. Interestingly, after cancers were becoming symphonized after the fifties of age, they are nowadays symphonized around the age of thirty years.

Analysis conducted revealed that heavy metals, such as lead and arsenic in pesticides, are concurrently found in cancer patients at considerably high levels.

Most people habitually drink polluted water. Such polluted water is considered a "time bomb" that results from the extremely high-poison pollution levels in the river water, which is righteously considered by scientists as one of the causes leading to cancer incidence.

So scientists recommend the use of an effective water filter with activated carbon layers. It is noteworthy that some mineral water bottles in the market are sometimes bottled from tap water.

Selenium element is considered one of the leading elements that play a vital role in conserving human health, as it was found that most cancer and heart diseases are in relation with soils containing low-selenium levels that result from pollution impacts. It has been scientifically confirmed that low-selenium inclusion levels are strangely associated with cancer and heart diseases.

And pursuant to a study conducted on 8,271 subjects for ten years, the U.S. Food Additives Center reported that intake of selenium has a cancer protective effect.

Life and Death of a Cancer Cell

The cancer cell is uniquely distinguished as being of self-growth, manipulated by gene-oriented directives more and above the cell's control potential. The alignment tumor herein reproduced is a more or less irregularly shaped mass, which attacks the normal tissues and eventually destroys them. If the cancer cells permeated the blood circulation, they thereby drift in the body and occupy distant destinations.

The body's baseline defense against tumors, as for defense against viruses and bacteria, is the immunity system syndrome. For unknown reasons, several tumors successfully removed from the white cells network fail to identify cancer cells as some foreign constituents in the body. If, however, the immune system could be activated for attack, it would thereby employ certain strategies, including those killing cells, that can devastate the cancer cells.

How Cancer Starts

No one knows exactly how cancer starts up. But what is clear is that it is triggered by genetic transformation. Such transformations activate the oncogenes, which exist in all human beings and cause natural genes to be affected with cancer. As a rule, oncogenes are habitually inert in natural genes.

How do oncogenes reproduce a carcinogenic cell? It is yet an unanswered question though that in some cases there are myriads of oncogenes to be activated. According to a potential scenario, the emitted ray that penetrates the cell shoots it and activates its embedded inert oncogene, termed proto-oncogenes.

The following step entails the interchange at strata within binary chromosomes, known as reciprocal translocation. One transformation is not harmful while the other is detrimental, as it reproduces a proto-oncogene adjacent to an active gene. This transformation activates another oncogene. In this case, the cell is unable to withstand these oncogenes, which results to a disfigured escaping tumor cell. That is the carcinogenic cell.

How Cancer Propagates

Metastasis is a process entailing the introduction of malignant cells into the bloodstream or the propagation of the lymphatic ducts throughout the body. This usually occurs virtually prior to diagnosing about half of the cancer cases. This is because secondary tumors are usually minute and escape before being discovered, leading to a delay in treatment.

In order that cancer cells can reach the blood, they secrete protein digestive enzymes that let them penetrate through the basic membrane. At that point, the cells associate with an alternating configuration protein (termed laminin) that causes further secretion of the said enzymes, which leads to the eruption of the basic membrane. This results to the exposure of protein cells that attract cancer cells.

Upon introduction of the carcinogenic cells into the bloodstream, they mostly dissipate, captured as victims of the natural killer cells transmitted by the immunity system. The remaining surviving cells dissipate toward an appropriate location in the brain or in the reproductive system where they penetrate the blood vessel wall, leading to the eruption of the basic diaphragm, then escaping into the tissues, where myriads of cellular layers rest in depth, settle and reproduce, resulting in secondary tumors; thus cancer propagation takes place.

The Increased Percentages of Cancer Diseases

Dr. Haddad's study pointed out to contracting 250,000 Egyptians with digestive system, rectum, and colon cancer diseases. The study, conducted by teamwork, carried out researches on cancer patients over an extended time period and revealed that the colon and rectum cancer patients in Egypt are mostly under thirty years of age, i.e., in their youth. This category is found in Egypt at a percentage exceeding that found in any other countries all over the world, knowing that this type of cancer has now become of first ranking position among males and females alike; after it was bladder cancer, which was first among males, and breast cancer, which was first among females.

In this study, it was noticed that there is a fourfold increase in the percentage of cancer diseases in Egypt over the past twenty years, which was more and above the previous percentage figures.

World Health Organization announced that a 50% increase is expected in cancer cases during the next twenty years.

Most of the cancer cases discovered nowadays result from continuous exposure to carcinogenic materials, rather than being due to a genes disorder.

The past twentieth century has provided us with the chemotherapy of cancer, so what should we expect to occur in the present twenty-first century? It has been confirmed that about two-thirds of the cancer cases may be avoided by modifying our daily lifestyles (smoking, alcoholic drinks, and nutrition). It has been statistically proven that it is possible to more likely avoid cancer than treat it.

Therefore, global research works are currently being conducted in view of minimizing cancer-catching cases, not by reducing exposure to carcinogenic materials, but through following a certain nutritional regimen.

Dr. Abdelfattah M. Badawi (1) and Dr. Manal M. Khowdiary (2)
(1), (2) Applied Surfactant Laboratory, Egyptian Petroleum Research Institute, Nasr City, Cairo, Egypt

Part One: Cancer Treatment by Orthomolecular Medicine

Chapter One: Selenium against Cancer

Chapter Two: Antioxidants against Cancer

Chapter Three: Vitamin C against Cancer

Part One

Cancer Treatment by Orthomolecular Medicine

Dr. Abdelfattah M. Badawi and Dr. Manal M. Khowdiary

ORTHOMOLECULAR MEDICINE IS the use of high doses of vitamins, minerals, or hormones to prevent and treat a wide variety of conditions. The doses are well above the recommended daily allowance (RDA) and may be used along with special diets and conventional treatments (1-3).

The use of large doses of nutrients for the treatment of cancer has not yet entered the mainstream of medicine, not in the universities, nor in the medical journals. But it is beginning to do so, largely due to the persistence and dedication of Prof. Linus Pauling (4).

During May 10-12, 1991, Jay Patrick, president of Alacer Corporation, hosted a meeting—the Second World Congress on Vitamin C and the Immune System—in San Diego. He had hosted the First World Congress on Vitamin C in 1978 in Palm Springs. That one was addressed by Dr. Szent-Gyorgyi, who won the Nobel

Prize for his work on vitamin C and intermediary metabolism, by Dr. Linus Pauling, and by Dr. Fred Klenner, the first physician to use megadoses of vitamin C. The Second World Congress brought together a distinguished group of vitamin researchers and clinicians including Dr. E. Cheraskin (5,6) and others.

Orthomolecular treatment improves the quality of life. It also decreases the side effects of radiation and chemotherapy. The program is palatable. The only patients who could not follow it were those who were getting chemotherapy and suffered severe nausea and vomiting or patients who could not swallow because of lesions in their throat. Orthomolecular therapy provides a step forward in the battle against cancer and must be fully explored. There can be no logical reason today why most of the research funds should go only toward the examination of more chemotherapy and more ways of giving radiation. There must be a major expansion into the use of orthomolecular therapy to sort out the variables and to determine how to improve the therapeutic outcome of treatment.

Vitamin Supplements

No one should take any supplements until they have become familiar with their properties and how to use them. It is advisable always to work with a knowledgeable physician. But if they cannot find any physician or orthomolecular nutritionist, they should go ahead on their own using the information now readily available on nutrition and vitamin supplements. They should advise their doctors what they are doing and which supplements they are using by listing the vitamins and dose ranges. I am not suggesting that every person needs to take them all. This is an individual matter based on discussions with his doctor whether the vitamins and mineral supplements are compatible with his medications and with his diet.

Vitamin C. The dose range is anywhere from three to forty grams daily in three divided doses. If the dose is too high, it will not be absorbed by the intestines and will stay in the bowel and act like a laxative causing loose stools and gas. It is a good laxative. The best dose does not act like a laxative. Forms of vitamin C include the pure ascorbic acid (hydrogen ascorbate) and the mineral salts, such as sodium ascorbate (slightly salty in taste), calcium ascorbate (slightly bitter), and other salts often found in combinations of the mineral ascorbates. In large doses, it is best used as the powder dissolved in water or one of the juices. Do not use commercial-grade vitamin C crystals or powders. Use CP grades as is found in drugstores or health food stores. Contrary to false rumors issued by some hostile critics of megadose vitamin use, it does not cause kidney stones, pernicious anemia, and sterility. A recent suggestion in a letter to *Nature*, published in England, concluded that more than 500 milligrams of vitamin C daily could cause DNA damage. This is based on one of twenty possible markers that could have been used, which showed no damage, and a twenty-first marker, which is seriously questioned. Some of the key scientists in this field criticized these conclusions. My only comment is that if they were correct, why do patients who take large doses of vitamin C live so much longer (7)?

Vitamin B3. There are two forms. Niacin lowers cholesterol, elevates high density lipoprotein cholesterol, and reduces the ravages of heart disease but causes flushing when it is first taken. The flushing reaction dissipates in time and, in most cases, is gone or very minor within a matter of weeks. Niacinamide, the other form, has no effect on blood fats (lipids) but is not a vasodilator. There have been seven international conferences on the theme *niacin and cancer*. This vitamin is an essential component of the enzyme systems that repair broken DNA molecules. The dose ranges from one hundred milligrams three times daily to one thousand milligrams three times daily. Several studies in Detroit have found that the response rate of cancer around the head and neck was 10% on radiation alone but increased to 80% when patients were given large doses of niacinamide (8).

Vitamin E (d-alpha tocopheryl succinate). This water-soluble form has the greatest efficacy in controlling cancer cell growth in the test tube and is the one I recommend should be used. The dose ranges from 400 to 1,200 International Units daily. Vitamin E is the major fat-soluble antioxidant in the body and plays a role by decreasing the concentration of free radicals, which are thought to be involved in the creation of the cancer. It also decreases the risk of heart disease, thus confirming what was found over fifty years in Ontario by Drs. Wilfrid and Evan Shute (9).

The Carotenoids. Most people have heard of beta-carotene, but this is only one of a large number of carotenoids which are present in colored vegetables and fruits, such as carrots, beets, tomatoes, and greens. The evidence is very powerful that these mixed carotenoids, as found in these foods, will decrease the incidence of cancer; but there is a question about the efficacy of the pure beta-carotene. There is still a vigorous debate about this. I prefer carrot juice for the beta-carotene. Generally, it is better to have a large variety of these natural anticancer factors. Beta-carotene is very safe. The only question is whether it is the best form. Only a small portion is converted into vitamin A.

Folic acid. Several studies have found this important vitamin has anticancer properties, for cancer of the cervix and of the lung in lung smokers. This does not mean it is safe to smoke. It does mean that smokers should take it and immediately start their campaign to stop smoking. Women should take ample amounts to prevent neural tube disorders such as spina bifida. The US government plans to add it to flour. Canada is still thinking about it. The dose range is from one to thirty milligrams daily. It can be taken only on prescription (10).

Coenzyme. Dr. Karl Folkers discovered this substance, also called ubiquinone; toward the end of his long and distinguished career, he regretted that he had not called it a vitamin. It is an odd vitamin since young people are able to make enough from the lower numbered ubiquinones, such as Q6 or Q8, whereas older people and anyone ill is not able to make enough. It thus becomes a vitamin later in life and when one becomes ill. A few clinical studies have shown that in large doses it has anticancer properties especially for breast cancer. These range from 300 milligrams to 600 milligrams daily.

Mineral Supplements

Selenium. The presence or absence of this trace element has the clearest relationship to the presence of cancer. People living on soils that are rich in selenium have a lower incidence. I recommend between 200 to 1,000 micrograms daily. One of my patients took 2,000 micrograms with no side effects.

Calcium and Magnesium. These are generally very useful to take to maintain calcium levels in bones and blood. They have been found helpful in cases of bowel cancer. Women should receive 1,500 milligrams of calcium daily from their food and supplements and half as much magnesium. There are several forms of these minerals available. Usually a person will absorb into their body anywhere between 25% and 50% of the calcium.

Zinc and Copper. There is a reciprocal connection between these two. If blood zinc levels are too high, the copper levels will be too low. Zinc can shrink enlarged prostate glands and may be helpful in the treatment of this cancer. I have been using it routinely. Also, people in Victoria tend to be low in zinc levels because their water is soft and dissolves copper more easily from copper plumbing.

Other Substances Found in Plants

A large number of these preparations are being used for the treatment of cancer. They include bioflavonoids, preparations from soybean and from mushrooms. Vaccines are also being used. Coley's vaccine originated over one hundred years ago. I will not discuss these, nor other treatments, such as 714-X, Ukrain, Iscador, Cartilage, Carnivora, Amygdalin (Laetrile), Essiac, and many herbs. These are described in the book by Diamond, Cowden, and Goldberg.

Most of the speakers at the 26th Annual International Conference on Nutritional Medicine Today, Toronto, April 1997, discussed various topics dealing with the principle and practice of orthomolecular medicine. Dr. C. Simone spoke on "Breast Cancer: Nutritional and Lifestyle Modification to Augment Oncology Care." Dr. Simone is well-known for his work in researching complementary treatment of cancer. He is an internist, medical oncologist, immunologist, and radiation oncologist and has published several valuable books including *Cancer & Nutrition: A Ten-Point Plan to Reduce Your Risk of Getting Cancer*. Optimum nutrition, avoiding toxic substances in food and water, and other lifestyle changes will materially reduce the risk of developing cancer.

Here is his ten-point plan: 1—Nutrition: calories slightly below average to maintain a weight just below the average weight. Should be high in fiber; rich in fish, fruits, and vegetables; and with vitamin and mineral supplements. Eliminate additives and salt. 2—Avoid tobacco. 3—Avoid alcohol (one drink per week allowed). 4—Avoid radiation. Take X-ray only when necessary and avoid excessive exposure to sun. 5—Keep environment, air, water, and workplace clean. 6—Avoid promiscuity, hormones, and any unnecessary drugs. 7—Learn early warning signs like a lump in the breast. 8—Exercise and relax regularly. 9—Take a yearly physical. 10—Read his book for a self-test of risk factors and symptoms that may indicate cancer or heart disease.

These ten points should be part of every treatment program as well. The main difference is that in treatment, the first point becomes even more important, and the doses of supplements are much greater. The sicker a person is, the more nutrients are needed in optimum doses to help the body's reparative mechanisms. Treatment must be started as soon as the diagnosis is suspected and made, and it should be concurrent with any other treatment recommended by oncologists and cancer specialists. Eventually, all cancer specialists will be using these orthomolecular techniques. Supplements must be maintained while chemotherapy or radiation is being used. Studies have shown that these supplements enhance the toxic effect of the treatment on the lesion and decrease the toxic effects on the body. Patients do not suffer as much from the side effects and recover much more quickly when the treatment series is completed. They enhance the quality of life during and after treatment.

There is no reason in the world why any oncologist should not allow vitamin treatment in combination with chemotherapy. This would enhance the therapeutic effect of the chemotherapy and would decrease its toxicity.

References

1. Versicherungsmedizin, Hakimi R. "[Prevention of metastasis with **orthomolecular** infusions and actovegin.]" 62(3), (September 1, 2010): 139-40. German.

2. Campos D., Austerlitz C., Allison RR, Póvoa H., Sibata C. "Nutrition and **orthomolecular** supplementation in lung **cancer** patients." *Integrative Cancer Therapies.* 8(4), (December 2009): 398-408.

3. McMichael A. J. "**Orthomolecular medicine** and megavitamin therapy." *Medical Journal of Australia.* 1(1), (January 10, 1981): 6-8.

4. Nature, Pauling L. **"Vitamins** and intelligence tests." 353(6340), (September 12, 1991): 103.

5. Cheraskin E. and Ringsdorf, WM Jr. "Predictive medicine." XV. Epilogue. *J. Am Geriatr Soc.* 20(4), (April 1972): 184-9.

6. Cheraskin, E. "Antioxidants in health and disease." *J. Am. Optom. Assoc.* 67(1), (January 1996): 50-7. Review.

7. Wróblewski K.Pol Merkur Lekarski. "[Can the administration of **large doses** of **vitamin C** have a harmful effect?]" 19(112), (October 2005): 600-3. Review. Polish.

8. Jackson TM, Rawling JM, Roebuck BD, Kirkland JB. **"Large** supplements of nicotinic acid and nicotinamide increase tissue NAD+ and poly(ADP-ribose) levels but do not affect diethylnitrosamine-induced altered hepatic foci in Fischer-344 rats." *J. Nutr.* 125(6), (June 1995): 1455-61.

9. Shute EV. "Treatment with **vitamin E**." *Can. Med. Assoc. J.* 22;107(2), (July 1972): 111.

10. Jägerstad M. **"Folic acid** fortification prevents neural tube defects and may also reduce **cancer** risks." *Acta Paediatr.* 101(10), (October 2012): 1007-12.

Chapter One
Selenium against Cancer

Dr. Abdelfattah M. Badawi and Dr. Manal M. Khowdiary

IT HAS BEEN recently proven that the rare element needed mostly by the body is the selenium element. Selenium is found in nature in the soil and in small quantities inside cereals, yeast, sesame seeds, garlic, mushroom, and fish.

Recent researches have revealed that selenium protects against hypertension and is an effective cure for blood circulation disturbances, as it is considered to be vital for the cardiac muscles. It is also effective against contacting the AIDS virus, the epidemic Hepatitis liver viruses, and malaria infection.

It has further more been noticed that high blood selenium levels is associated with lower percentage of cancer cases. The great majority of people don't get their need of selenium even though they may be consuming foods rich in this element. This element may be considered the most important among trace elements as it assumes a vital role in human health.

In this regard, all kinds of cancers, including leukemia, besides various cardiac diseases may be due to the deficiency of selenium levels in the human body. Reduced levels of selenium are always associated with high percentage cases of cardiac diseases and cancer, particularly breast cancer. Accordingly, foods with high content of selenium could significantly reduce the risks of catching cancer.

The powerful cancer protective effects provided by selenium are due to the composition of this element (superoxide anions). It has been noticed that selenium kills the human cancer cells at a 55% percentage within seventy-two hours; and this element, moreover, reduces lung cancer cells, as well as it reduces the growth rate of liver cancer cells and human brain cancer cells.

Dr. Shruzer, professor of chemistry in California University, carried out experiments on a set of breast cancer—susceptible rats. It was noticed that the set of rats not having consumed sufficient selenium percentages developed breast cancer at a rate of 83% compared with the set of rats whose food selenium percentage content was high and developed only 10% breast cancer cases.

Dr. Shruzer discovered, as a result of many of his experiments, that the higher the selenium percentages in human food, the less likely one becomes prone to catch cancer. Reduced levels of selenium in the human blood are usually associated with an increased potential to catch cancer so that the animals which are exposed to carcinogenic materials and consume large quantities of selenium are the least to catch cancer.

In the Hospital of London's department of clinical pharmacology, test animals were dosed simultaneously with carcinogenic materials and selenium. After twelve months, it was noticed that the percent occurrence of cancer in those animals decreased from 82% to 48% in the group of animals which consumed 2 ppm selenium and down to 12% in the group which consumed 6 ppm of selenium. Moreover, experiments have confirmed that the selenium that is added to the food stops the occurrence of breast cancer, which is evoked by carcinogenic materials.

In about twenty-seven countries worldwide, it has been established that the selenium level in food is inversely proportional with the occurrence of cancer cases, particularly breast, ovary, colon, and rectum cancers and leukemia. Knowing that blood selenium levels in the citizens of seventeen countries were inversely proportional to the rates of breast cancer cases and with every increase in the soil's natural selenium percentage content in these countries, the number of cancer-catching cases lessened. In countries whose natives consume high doses of selenium, they are accompanied with reduced death cases resulting from leukemia and stomach, rectum, prostate, breast, ovary, lung, pancreas, skin, and bladder cancers.

In China, for instance, it was noticed that in the southern zones there is evidence that liver cancers are widespread, surpassing those occurring in the northern zones. By analyzing the selenium percentage contents in either zones' crops, it was observed that such selenium contents were markedly lower in the southern zones.

It was also found that in Europe, the rate of catching cancer is proportional to the biologically available selenium. In Finland, the selenium content level was measured in the bloods of 8,000 noncancer men and women over a five-year period, whence the final results confirmed that the persons who had caught cancer were those whose blood selenium content level was low.

Whereas in Eastern Asia (Japan, Thailand, and the Philippines), analysis have shown that the selenium percentage content (0.26-0.29 ppm), which is accounted to be a high percentage content, was attributed with lower rates of breast cancer cases (0.8-8.5 cases among every 100,0000 persons).

On the other hand, in the USA, citizens of fifty-five years of age and above constituted 90% of the cancer cases, which amount to 1.3 million new cancer cases annually in accordance to the following findings:

The blood selenium content levels approximately 0.07 ppm, which is actually a low-percentage level was associated with

- a high percentage of breast cancer cases (nineteen to twenty-two cases) in every 100,000.

- a high percentage of lung cancer (thirty-seven cases) in every 100,000.

We might conclude from the foregoing that the key element in self-protection against cancer lies in consuming the sufficient amount of the selenium element, knowing that those persons susceptible to cancer due to the a family heredity trend or those employed in chemical or metalworking industries should benefit from increasing selenium content in their diet in order to avoid catching cancer.

An interesting study was carried out in China on 20,000 persons in a certain city, who were susceptible to liver cancer, and selenium was added to the table salt at a 5.6 ppm. It was compared with another sector of people of 110,000 persons consuming selenium-free table salt.

And after the lapse of five years, it was found that the city dwellers who had selenium added to their diet's salt recorded percentage rates of catching liver cancer 43% less than was the case for the other city dwellers whose diet's table salt devoid of selenium added.

Also, in another study carried out on 2,474 persons whose families were subject to liver cancer, one group consumed 2,000 micrograms selenium daily, compared to a group that didn't consume this element. The results were amazing, as the liver cancer cases percentage was reduced at 45% in comparison with the persons who didn't consume the selenium element. This was statistically confirmed to be 95%.

And in the USA, 8,274 persons were subjected to the test during a period of ten years (1983-1993) in a pioneering experience initiated by the Nutritional Prevention of Cancer (NPC) in which the elderly were treated with 200 micrograms selenium daily; whence the following was noticed.

It was concluded from these experiments that selenium has a protective action against cancer by virtue of activating activity of the selenoproteins in the human body, which have a protective effect against free radicals.

In the United States, it was proved that high levels of zinc are associated with reduction of the blood selenium percentage content, which indicates that consuming given doses of zinc obstructs the adsorption of the selenium element, besides the fact that vitamin C impedes the protective impact of selenium against cancer, as vitamin C converts selenium compounds (selenite) to the water-insoluble selenium element and which is consequently not absorbed or nutritionally assimilated.

On the other hand, vitamin E and vitamin A promote the effectiveness of selenium in cancer protection. Experts recommend administering vitamin C in the morning, while administering selenium combined with vitamin E and vitamin A at night, without administration of any other vitamins or minerals that impede the adsorption of selenium possessing cancer protection impact.

In this concern, the most recent global clinical research works carried out in Australia, published in 2004, confirmed that consuming high doses of the selenium element promotes impeding the widespread of prostate cancer.

The Scientific Gynecological Oncology Journal of Poland published in 2004 an article reporting that consuming selenium element in conjunction with chemotherapy has a supporting influence in treating ovary cancer cases.

In China, the journal *Progress in Chemistry* published in 2004 that the biological function of selenium in preventing cancer can be explained by inducing apoptosis of tumor cells. This is an interdisciplinary frontier of the bioinorganic chemistry of selenium and its related subjects, and the journal *Colloids and Surfaces* published in 2011 a simple method for fabrication of sialic acid surface-decorated selenium nanoparticles (SA-Se-NPs), with enhanced cancer-targeting and cell-penetrating abilities that was demonstrated in the present study. Monodisperse and homogeneous spherical SA-Se-NPs with striking stability were prepared under the optimized conditions. SA surface decoration significantly increased the cellular uptake and cytotoxicity of Se-NPs in HeLa human cervical carcinoma cells. Treatments of SA-Se-NPs induced dose-dependent apoptosis in HeLa cells, as evidenced by increase in sub-G1 cell populations, nuclear condensation, and formation of apoptotic bodies.

The American journal *Nanomedicine: Nanotechnology, Biology, and Medicine* reported the synthesis of stable selenium nanoparticles (SeNPs) and the elucidation of their mechanism of action in preventing the growth of mammary tumors. Cell viability and expression of apoptotic markers (pp38, Bax, and cytochrome c) were assessed in MCF-7 and MDA-MB-231 breast cancer cells treated with SeNPs. Reduction in tumor volume was measured in rats; interestingly, animals showing significant decrease in tumor volume (small tumors) had lower levels of ERα as compared with animals showing a nonsignificant decrease in tumor volume (large tumor). This is the first report in our knowledge suggesting that the anticancer activity of SeNPs correlates with the size of breast cancer cells both in vivo and in vitro (1).

The journal *Biomaterials* recently reported that antiangiogenesis is an effective strategy for cancer treatment because uncontrolled tumor growth depends on tumor angiogenesis and sufficient blood supply. Thus, blocking angiogenesis could be a strategy to arrest tumor growth. The function and mechanism of luminescent ruthenium-modified selenium nanoparticles (Ru-SeNPs) in angiogenesis have not been elucidated to date. Here, they found that Ru-SeNPs significantly inhibited human umbilical vascular endothelial cell (HUVEC) proliferation, migration, and tube formation. Ru-SeNPs was also tested in vivo in the chicken chorioallantoic membrane (CAM) assay and found to inhibit bFGF-treated CAMs development like suramin. Moreover, we showed that Ru-SeNPs inhibited the activations of FGFR1 and its downstream protein kinases. Furthermore, by using fluorescence confocal microscopy and TEM imaging studies, we have demonstrated their cellular uptake and localization within the cytoplasm of HepG2 and HUVEC cells. These findings indicate that Ru-SeNPs inhibits angiogenesis and may be a viable drug candidate in antiangiogenesis and anticancer therapies (2).

The American journal *Cancer Research* recently reported that selenium exists in a number of forms with differing valence states, some of which have shown antitumor activity. Four currently available selenium forms were studied for their tumoricidal activity against a human leukemia cell line and exploited the differences among them to investigate the mechanism of antitumor action. Only selenocystine and sodium selenite showed antitumor activity, and these were also the only compounds which demonstrated significant redox chemistry, including depletion of cellular glutathione, stimulation of glutathione reductase, and stimulation of oxygen consumption. The interaction of these two compounds with glutathione suggests an intriguing potential role for them in cancer therapy (3).

The *Russian Journal of Physical Chemistry* recently reported that nanostructures formed during the reduction of ionic selenium in the selenite-ascorbate redox system in an aqueous solution of bovine serum albumin (BSA) were studied using static and dynamic light scattering and flow birefringence. It was established that this process results in the formation of stable aggregates of selenium nanoparticles that adsorb BSA molecules. It was found that highly ordered super high-molecular weight spherical nanostructures with high density and unique morphology are formed. Experiments with a cell culture of promyelocytic leukemia HL-60 showed that BSA adsorbed on selenium nanoparticles can inhibit the growth of tumor cells and deactivate free radicals with an efficiency comparable with that of sodium selenite (4).

Advanced Science Letters, American scientific publishers, indicated that the specific anticarcinogenic properties of Se and the phloroglucinol ones have coupled in new amorphous Se nanoparticles, surface capped with phloroglucinol synthesized in mild conditions, which may be used in biomedical field. The phloroglucinol surface protected Se nanoparticles have been synthesized according to a new green method without any organic solvent and using phloroglucinol as reducing and capping agent in order to obtain Se nanoparticles suitable for interesting anticancer biomedical applications (5).

In China, the journal *Biomaterials* reported that the study of a novel organoselenium compounds that induce apoptosis of human oral squamous cell carcinoma Tca83. Human oral squamous cell carcinoma Tca83 were cultured in a medium, which were treated with the novel organoselenium compounds with different doses. The survival rates of cells were calculated by apoptotic flow cytometer after twenty-four hours. Results indicated that the novel organoselenium compounds induced apoptosis, and the apoptotic rates increased with the adding of doses, and every groups had obvious differences. This indicated that these novel organoselenium compounds induced apoptosis, and the apoptotic rates depended on the doses (6).

Nanomedicine: Nanotechnology, Biology, and Medicine journal reported a simple method for preparation of adenosine triphosphate (ATP) surface-functionalized selenium nanoparticles (SeNPs@ ATP) with enhanced cell permeabilization and anticancer activity. Spherical SeNPs were decorated with ATP by strong adsorption through an Se-N bond, leading to the highly stable structure of the conjugates. ATP surface decoration significantly enhanced the cellular uptake and anticancer activity of SeNPs. Induction of apoptosis in human hepatocellular carcinoma cells by SeNPs@ATP was evidenced by accumulation of the sub-Group 1 cell population, phosphatidylserine exposure, DNA fragmentation, PARP cleavage and caspase activation. Further studies found that SeNPs@ATP treatment triggered the depletion of mitochondrial membrane potential and reactive oxygen species (ROS) overproduction. These results demonstrated that the use of ATP as a surface decorator of SeNPs is a novel strategy to achieve anticancer synergy. SeNPs@ATP may be a candidate for further evaluation as a chemotherapeutic agent for human cancers (7).

Bioscience, Biotechnology, and Biochemistry journal reported the estimation of the nutritional availability of selenium (Se) in selenium-enriched Kaiware radish sprouts (SeRS) by the tissue Se deposition and glutathione peroxidase (GPX) activity of rats administered the sprouts and examined the effect of SeRS on the formation of aberrant crypt foci (ACF) in the colon of mice administered 1,2-dimethylhydrazine (DMH) to evaluate antitumor activity. Male weanling Wistar rats were divided into seven groups and fed a Se-deficient basal diet or the basal diet supplemented with 0.05, 0.10, or 0.15 µg/g of Se as sodium selenite or SeRS for twenty-eight days. Supplementation with Se dose dependently increased serum and liver Se concentrations and GPX activities, and the selenite-supplemented groups showed a higher increase than the SeRS-supplemented groups. The nutritional availability of Se in SeRS was estimated to be thirty-three or 64% by slope ratio analysis. Male four-week-old A/J mice were divided into seven groups and fed a low-Se basal diet or the basal diet supplemented with selenite, SeRS, or selenite plus non-Se-enriched radish sprouts (NonSeRS) at a level of 0.1 or 2.0 µg Se/g for nine weeks. After one week of feeding, all mice were given six subcutaneous injections of DMH (20 mg/kg) at one-week intervals. The average number of ACF formed in the colon of mice fed the basal diet was 4.3. At a supplementation level of 0.1 µg Se/g, only SeRS significantly inhibited ACF formation. At a supplementation level of 2.0 µg Se/g, both selenite and SeRS significantly inhibited ACF formation. The addition of NonSeRS to the selenite-supplemented diets tended to inhibit ACF formation, but this was not statistically significant. These results indicate that SeRS shows lower nutritional availability but higher antitumor activity than selenite (8).

The journal *Biological Trace Element Research* reported that selenium is a trace element that is essential to the human diet. Deficiency states have been described in both animals and humans.

In addition, selenium compounds have demonstrated toxicity in humans, as well as in human tissues in culture. As early as 1956, one form of selenium was used as an antineoplastic agent in humans with some demonstrated activity. Recently, evidence in both tumor-bearing animals and human tumor cells in culture have confirmed an antitumor effect of potential clinical benefit. The mechanism of this cytotoxic effect appears, at least in part, to relate to the property of some forms of selenium to oxidize critical sulfhydryl groups in the cells. Evidence for this, and the resulting implications for the use of selenium in anticancer treatment, is presented in this journal (9).

ACS Nano reported a simple method for preparing 5-fluorouracil surface-functionalized selenium nanoparticles (5FU-SeNPs) with enhanced anticancer activity has been demonstrated. Spherical SeNPs were capped with 5FU through formation of Se-O and Se-N bonds and physical adsorption, leading to the stable structure of the conjugates. 5FU surface decoration significantly enhanced the cellular uptake of SeNPs through endocytosis. A panel of five human cancer cell lines was shown to be susceptible to 5FU-SeNPs, with IC50 values ranging from 6.2 to 14.4 μM. Despite this potency, 5FU-SeNP possesses great selectivity between cancer and normal cells. Induction of apoptosis in A375 human melanoma cells by 5FU-SeNPs was evidenced by accumulation of sub-G1 cell population, DNA fragmentation, and nuclear condensation. The contribution of the intrinsic apoptotic pathway to the cell apoptosis was confirmed by activation of caspase-9 and depletion of mitochondrial membrane potential. Pretreatment of cells with a general caspase inhibitor z-VAD-fmk significantly prevented 5FU-SeNP-induced apoptosis, indicating that 5FU-SeNP induced caspase-dependent apoptosis in A375 cells. Furthermore, 5FU-SeNP-induced apoptosis was found dependent on ROS generation. Our results suggest that the strategy to use SeNPs as a carrier of 5FU could be a highly efficient way to achieve anticancer synergism. 5FU-SeNPs may be a candidate for further evaluation as a chemo preventive and chemotherapeutic agent for human cancers, especially melanoma (10).

In China, the journal *Inorganic Chemistry* reported that surface charge plays a key role in cellular uptake and biological actions of nanomaterials. Selenium nanoparticles (SeNPs) are novel Se species with potent anticancer activity and low toxicity. This study constructed positively charged SeNPs by chitosan surface decoration to achieve selective cellular uptake and enhanced anticancer efficacy. The results of structure characterization revealed that hydroxyl groups in chitosan reacted with SeO_3^{2-} ion to form special chain-shaped intermediates, which could be decomposed to form crystals upon reduction by ascorbic acid. The initial colloids nucleated and then assembled into spherical SeNPs. The positive charge of the NH_3^+ group on the outer surface of the nanoparticles contributed to the high stability in aqueous solutions. Moreover, a panel of four human cancer cell lines was found to be susceptible to SeNPs, with IC50 values ranging from 22.7 to 49.3 µM. Chitosan surface decoration of SeNPs significantly enhanced the selective uptake by endocytosis in cancer cells and thus amplified the anticancer efficacy. Treatment of the A375 melanoma cells with chitosan—SeNPs led to dose-dependent apoptosis, as evidenced by DNA fragmentation and phosphatidylserine translocation (11).

Biological Trace Element Research reported that selenium salts as well as elemental selenium nanoparticles are attracting the attention of researchers due to their excellent biological properties. The aim of this work was to study immunomodulation by applying elemental SeNPs to stimulate the immune response of mice bearing breast cancer tumors. Six- to eight-week-old female inbred mice were divided into two groups of test and control, each containing fifteen mice. Every day, for two weeks prior to tumor induction, selenium nanoparticles were orally administered to the mice at a dose of 100 µg/day. Then, 1×10^6 cells from a breast cancer tumors cell line were injected subcutaneously to each mouse. Oral nanoparticle administration was continued daily for three weeks after tumor induction. Different immunological parameters were then evaluated including cytokine level, delayed type hypersensitivity (DTH) response as well as tumor growth and the survival rates in all treated or nontreated animals. The DTH response of test mice also showed a significant increase when compared to the control mice. The survival rate was notably higher for the selenium nanoparticle-treated mice compared to the control mice (12).

Molecular Nutrition and Food Research reported that prostate cancer (PC) chemoprevention has generated considerable interest in the last decade, and selenium and combinations of selenium have been recognized as one of the most efficacious chemopreventive agents against PC. This review focuses on a discussion of the knowledge hitherto gained about the mechanisms of action of the various in vitro- and in vivo-used selenium compounds and their effects on cellular processes and signaling pathways. This paper also describes the clinical and preclinical studies that have contributed enormously to the knowledge about dose, duration of exposure, and the chemical form of selenium effective in different scenarios. Even though the jury is still out about whether selenium can be used as a chemopreventive agent in the clinic and whether studies with cell lines and populations at low, medium, or high risk can adequately represent the physiological behavior of this micronutrient, it can safely be said to offer the most diverse spectrum of protective effects against this particular type of cancer which may augur well for its future as a chemopreventive agent (13).

References

1. Jun-Sheng Zheng, Shan-Yuan Zheng, Yi-Bo Zhang, Bo Yu, Wenjie Zheng, Fang Yang, Tianfeng Chen. "Sialic acid surface decoration enhances cellular uptake and apoptosis-inducing activity of selenium nanoparticles." Vol. 83 (2011): 183-187.

2. Dongdong Sun, Yanan Liu, Qianqian Yu, Yanhui Zhou, Rong Zhang, Xiaojia Chen, An Hong, Jie Liu. "The effects of luminescent ruthenium(II) polypyridyl functionalized selenium nanoparticles on bFGF-induced angiogenesis and AKT/ERK signaling." *Biomaterials*. Vol. 34, Issue 1 (2013): 171-180.

3. Gerald Batist1, Aspandiar G. Katki, Raymond W. Klecker Jr., and Charles E. Myers. "Selenium-induced Cytotoxicity of Human Leukemia Cells: Interaction with Reduced Glutathione." *Cancer Res*. 46 (1986): 5482.

4. S. V. Valueva, L. N. Borovikova, V. V. Koreneva, Ya. I. Nazarkina, A. I. Kipper, V. V. Kopeikin. "Structural-morphological and biological properties of selenium nanoparticles stabilized by bovine serum albumin." *Russian Journal of Physical Chemistry*. Vol. 81, 7 (2007): 1170-1173.

5. Fracasso, G.; Foresti, E.; Lesci, I.G.; Roveri, N. "Synthetic Phloroglucinol Surface Protected Se Nanoparticles for Potential Biomedical Applications." Vol. 4, Number 2, (2011): 610-61.

6. ZHANG Lei, CHANG Huai-guang, WANG Zhi-ying. "The Study of a Novel Organoselenium Compounds (Eb) Inducing Apoptosis of Human Oral Squamous Cell Carcinoma Tca83 in Vitro." *Biomaterials*. Vol. 34, Issue 1 (January 2013): 171-180

7. Yibo Zhang MS, Xiaoling Li, Zhi Huang, Wenjie Zheng, Cundong Fan, Tianfeng Chen. "Enhancement of cell permeabilization apoptosis-inducing activity of selenium nanoparticles by ATP surface decoration, Nanotechnology." *Biology and Medicine*. Volume 9, Issue 1 (2013): 74-84.

8. Fukunaga K, Matsuzaki Y, Yoshida M, Namikawa Y, Nishiyama T, Okada T. "Evaluation of Nutritional Availability and Anti-Tumor Activity of Selenium Contained in Selenium-Enriched Kaiware Radish Sprouts." *Bioscience, Biotech. and Biochemistry*. Vol. 71, No. 9 (2007) 2198-2205.

9. Batist, Gerald. "Selenium, Biological Trace Element Research." 1988, Volume 15, Issue 1, (1988): 223-229.

10. Wen Liu, Xiaoling Li, Yum-Shing Wong, Wenjie Zheng, Yibo Zhang, Wenqiang Cao and Tianfeng Chen. "Selenium Nanoparticles as a Carrier of 5-Fluorouracil to Achieve Anticancer Synergism." *ACS Nano*. 6 (8). 2012.

11. Bo Yu, Yibo Zhang, Wenjie Zheng, Cundong Fan, and Tianfeng Chen. "Positive Surface Charge Enhances Selective Cellular Uptake and Anticancer Efficacy of Selenium Nanoparticles." *Inorg. Chem.*, 51 (16), (2012): 8956-8963.

12. Mohammad Hossein Yazdi, Mehdi Mahdavi, Bardia Varastehmoradi, Mohammad Ali Faramarzi, Ahmad Reza Shahverdi. "The Immunostimulatory Effect of Biogenic Selenium Nanoparticles on the 4T1 Breast Cancer Model: an In Vivo Study." Volume 149, Issue 1, (October 2012): 22-28.

13. Gao, Allen C. "Mechanisms of selenium chemoprevention and therapy in prostate cancer Nagalakshmi Nadiminty." Volume 52, Issue 11 (2008): 1247-1260.

Chapter Two
Antioxidants against Cancer

Dr. Abdelfattah M. Badawi and Dr. Manal M. Khowdiary

What Could Be the Cancer Protective Means?

THIS QUESTION IS posed by many people who have contracted cancer, as well as by those who have observed their striving relatives and friends this invalidity. This question is set forth by people from all classes, occupations, and age brackets. And cancer is frightful and costly as it disrupts and destroys the lives of those suffering therefrom; in all families no one's having any immunity therefrom.

Good news has surfaced resulting from the scientific research works that have succeeded over the last ten years to establish the possibility for individuals to reduce the risks inherent in many types of cancer.

The key to reducing the risks lies in appropriate nutrition and resorting to the right food additive and avoiding carcinogenic materials and improving the standards of living. This is upon knowing that the different environmental factors constitute even up to 70% of all types of cancer and carcinogenic materials which result from genetic disorder which can be duly controlled by means of antioxidants.

What is the Possible Means in Order to Mitigate Side Effects of Surgery, Radioactivity, and Chemical Therapy?

Invalids want indeed to mitigate the destructive effects they suffer and which attack the blood and the spine, leading to losing hair and mouth inflammation and many of the ill effects which render radiology and chemical therapy an unsustainable nightmare.

In this regard, scientists firmly believe that antioxidants can be administered to those patients under traditional radiological and chemical therapies. Antioxidants can prove to be most effective factors in mitigating undesirable side effects. And upon the cancer patients having completed their traditional therapy, there arises a question mark, as to whether there is a possibility for expediting their recovery; the answer being yes, for antioxidants have capacities to activate the secondary latent in the human body power. In addition to an endeavor to improve the daily diet routine, patients should give up smoking and harmful intake while increasing their corporal activity by packing sports and avoiding X-rays and maintaining an optimistic state of mind. All these factors are of utmost importance in view of avoiding cancer.

The term "antioxidant" goes back to the year 1920 and refers to any substance that resists oxidation and other forms of oxidation. Oxygen-containing compounds generate molecules termed "free radicals." In the body, these free radicals trigger chain reactions. Scientific findings during the recent few decades have indicated that free radicals can destroy the gene matter ousting them from the fats or from the proteins, knowing that there is a belief that is liable for many of old-age traits and many diseases such as cancer. And even cancers believed to be reproduced pursuant to mechanical factors (e.g., exposure to asbestos) have been proven nowadays to be produced by free radical constituents.

And during the last decade, it has been proven that antioxidants play a significant role in any anticancer program. And besides the diet program, which depends on the outcoming system, antioxidants may be considered the first and most powerful line of defense against all types of cancer.

There are thousands of scientific articles referring to the power inherent in antioxidants. And many doctors are unaware of such power in their course of college study of medicine, and other doctors may by knowledgeable about the fantastic development oncoming antioxidants; but mostly these scientists, including the doctors, endorse the positive reports about food additives.

Scientific researches about antioxidants are promising, although there isn't sufficient information leading to decisive results.

Dr. Richard Horton, editor-in-chief of *The Lancet* medical magazine in 1959.

However, in spite of focusing on cancer, antioxidants are most important in the protection against heart attacks, clots, and eyeball dissociation besides a hundred diseases associated with old age. Here one becomes aware of the relevant reason underlying the necessity of his daily diet being of high antioxidants and food additives content.

We should also perceive that antioxidants are but a single facet of the complete picture pertaining to avoiding cancer.

As there are other facets that comprise herbs, fatty acids, algae, and mushroom whose beneficial effect is by virtue of the antioxidants' activity; only a few people receive the sufficient daily needs of fruits and vegetables. Moreover, a total deficiency in the vital nutritional elements in baby foods shall affect their future as well as affecting our society. It has now been quite clear that food additives are most necessary in view of the protection against cancer as well as against other diseases. In this regard, the US Medical Institute of the National Academy for Sciences has advocated since 1998 the significance of administrating folic acid and vitamin B12. It has also been increasingly recommended to note the importance of administering vitamin C and E on a daily basis. And nowadays, the US Medical Society's journal, as well as other medical journals, also advocate the importance of taking in high doses of these vitamins.

The College of Food Science and Technology, Nanjing Agricultural University in China reported the antioxidant and antitumor activities (in vitro) of superfine regular and Se-enriched green tea particles with different sizes (3.52 µm and 220 nm). The vitamin C and tea polyphenol contents of green tea in different sizes were significantly different, and amino acid and chlorophyll just changed a little. The antioxidant activity of green tea particles was evaluated by radical scavenging and linoleic acid peroxidation inhibition methods, and the antitumor activity was evaluated by ant proliferation assay on liver (HepG2), lung A (549), and myeloma gastric MGC803 tumor cells. The results indicated that enrichment of selenium endowed green tea with higher antioxidant activity and antitumor activity on HepG2 and A549 tumor cells. The radical scavenging rates of regular and Se-enriched green tea of 220 nm (67.87% and 69.49%, respectively) were significantly greater than that of 3.52 µm, but the inhibition of linoleic acid peroxidation for green tea of 220 nm was lower. The inhibitory rates of green tea of 220 nm on HepG2, A549, and MGC803 cells achieved 77.35%, 80.76%, and 87.54% for regular green tea, and 82.51%, 88.09%, and 74.48% for Se-enriched green tea at the dose of 100 µg mL-1, values that were all significantly higher compared to that of 3.52 µm (1).

Antioxidants As a Cancer-Curing Means:

There are some patients who attempt to identity alternative cancer-curing means after the unsuccessful outcomes of the traditional ways. Some thereof seek to avoid surgery, radiology, and chemical therapy.

There are numerous cases of some people who have resorted to super high antioxidant doses and who have been able to realize a retreat in their cancer tumors, knowing that a great number of experts rely on antioxidants as part of the untraditional curing program, such airing means being promising, yet not duly confirmed.

Much of these curing means are independent from the programs, established by Dr. Linus Pauling, twice Nobel Prize holder. That program was implemented by his Scottish colleague, Dr. Ian Cameron, whence these therapy trials were tested in the Mayo Clinic Hospital.

We shall make reference in the course of this book to positive clinical human tests, which comprise several studies related to administering high dose groups of antioxidant in association with the BCG serum in airing bladder cancer.

Concurrently, clinical trails have been undertaken in view of extracting high antioxidant doses and which regulated in highly positive results. And Dr. David Lamb and his colleagues of the west Bees a College of Medicine treated sixty-five bladder cancer patients resorting to a traditional airing means termed BCG, whence thirty patients were administered reduced antioxidant doses while thirty-five patients were administered high doses of the following food additives:

Type of food Additive	Daily Dose
Vitamin C	2000 milligrams
Vitamin A	$40,000 \pm$ milligrams
Vitamin B_6	100 milligrams
Vitamin E	40 milligrams
Zinc	90 milligrams

Usually bladder cancer recurs symphonizing after the lapse of ten months; at the start of the program, recurrence of the cancer symptom in the group that was administered with high food additives started to retreat. Five years later, the rate of retreat in the group having been administered high food additive doses is found to be at a 41% rate compared to a 91% retreat rate for those that were administered low food additive doses.

Reference

1. Huajia Li, Feng Li, Fangmei Yang, Yong Fang, Zhihong Xin, Liyan Zhao, and Qiuhui Hu. "Size Effect of Se-Enriched Green Tea Particles on in vitro Antioxidant and Antitumor Activities." *J. Agric. Food Chem.*, 56 (12), (2008): 4529-4533.

Chapter Three
Vitamin C against Cancer

Dr. Abdelfattah M. Badawi and Dr. Manal M. Khowdiary

Dr. MCCORMICK IS considered as among the first ones who recorded that the ones suffering from cancer have very low levels of vitamin C, and he noticed that the symptoms of the lack of vitamin C disease, which is the scurvy disease, are similar to some types of blood cancers (leukemia) and also other types of cancer (1).

Dr. McCormick discovered that the main effort against cancer should aim to prevent it from spreading in the body as the result of cellular division. He suggested the use of vitamin C as the cellular tearing depends on the weakness of the connective tissue, and vitamin C strengthens it and prevents its division. A simple hypothesis target was the treatment basis for Dr. Linus Pauling, who received the Nobel Prize twice and who pointed elaborately about this in his book *Cancer and Vitamin C*. He recorded about the use of high doses of vitamin C and that the cancerous cells try to spread in the body, and they are prevented by vitamin C that strengthens the collagen and the connective tissues and prevents their division. Dr. Pauling announced that the high doses of vitamin C could be considered as similar to an antibiotic as they are working against viruses or bacteria, and they assist the immunity system; and even the arterial sclerosis, which is the main cause of the heart diseases, is imputed to the deficiency in vitamin C (2).

Dr. Pauling confirmed that the cancer patients can live longer and even can be cured with sufficient doses of vitamin C.

An intravenous injection of a dose of vitamin C (5 grams) in a patient's body is sufficient for killing the pathological microbes in this patient's body, as Dr. Pauling stated. The wild gorilla eats plants daily, containing 4.5 grams of vitamin C. The primitive man was a vegetarian, and his daily intake of vitamin C amounted to 2.3 to 9.5 grams. Dr. Erwin Stone confirmed the scientific fact that the human being needs high doses of vitamin C for protecting himself from the microbes' infection and stress.

Dr. Linus used the comparative biochemistry for confirming the fact of the high requirement for vitamin C, and he named the new treatment as the "Orthomolecular Medicine." And as one of the greatest scientists, Dr. Linus was happy when he was named "the vitamin C man."

Are the high doses of vitamin C safe?

Vitamin C is a simple molecule used by animals and plants in high doses; therefore this vitamin is considered as safe in high doses and for long periods without any harm, and it is a very safe compound more than any other medicines (3).

Cancer and vitamin C

The life expectancy averages have increased and consequently the cancer infliction, and therefore one of every three persons has a possibility of being inflicted by this disease usually at the later years of life, and consequently it was very important to understand how and why the cancer evolves.

The essential role of vitamin C and the other antioxidants for the protection against cancer has recently become very apparent, and the governing critical factors for the cell division is the availability of vitamin C. High doses of vitamin C with other nutritive complements have the ability to prevent cancer and even to treat it. It was proven that the acute deficiency in vitamin C and other antioxidants may cause the cell to grow and divide; this is what is known as "cancer." The high doses of vitamin C support the processes of oxidation, reduction, and immunity; and that's what stands behind the auto recovery.

It was noticed that the leukemia patients were suffering from a deficiency in vitamin C; and from Dr. William McCormick's point of view, there is a relation between the cancer disease and the deficiency of vitamin C, as cancer is a disease that is distinguished by the deficiency of collagen resulting from the deficiency of vitamin C. It was proven that high doses of vitamin C are poisonous for the malignant cancerous cells. This was confirmed by the researches of Dr. Erwin Stone, who proved the existence of a relation between the deficiency of vitamin C and cancer.

There is a study about a patient who was suffering from leukemia, and he was treated daily with doses of 24-42 grams of vitamin C. When the patient stopped twice the intake of vitamin C, his condition deteriorated; and when the treatment was resumed with high doses of vitamin C, the cancer retreated, and he was cured by this treatment system. Dr. Pauling recorded that the patients who are treated with this system lived in average five times longer than the patients who were not treated with this system.

Many recent researches point that the processes of oxidation and reduction that depend on vitamin C have a great importance for the protection from cancer. Early clinical studies showed that high-dose vitamin C, given by intravenous and oral routes, may improve symptoms and prolong life in patients with terminal cancer. Recent evidence shows that oral administration of the maximum tolerated dose of vitamin C (18 grams/day) produces peak plasma concentrations of only 220 µmol/L, whereas intravenous administration of the same dose produces plasma concentrations about twenty-fivefold higher. Larger doses (50-100 g) given intravenously may result in plasma concentrations of about 14,000 µmol/L. At concentrations above 1000 µmol/L, vitamin C is toxic to some cancer cells but not to normal cells in vitro. We found three well-documented cases of advanced cancers, confirmed by histopathologic review, where patients had unexpectedly long survival times after receiving high-dose intravenous vitamin C therapy. We examined clinical details of each case in accordance with National Cancer Institute (NCI) Best Case Series guidelines. Tumor pathology was verified by pathologists at the NCI who were unaware of diagnosis or treatment. In light of recent clinical pharmacokinetic findings and in vitro evidence of antitumor mechanisms, these case reports indicate that the role of high-dose intravenous vitamin C therapy in cancer treatment should be reassessed.

Six men and six women consumed 500 mL commercial fresh-squeezed orange juice/day for fourteen days, corresponding to an intake of 250 mg ascorbic acid/day. On the first day of the study, the subjects drank the juice in one dose (dose-response study), and on days 2-14 they consumed 250 mL in the morning and 250 mL in the afternoon. Blood was collected every hour for six hours on the first day and again on days 7 and 14. Baseline plasma vitamin C concentrations were significantly higher ($P = 0.03$) among the women than among the men (56.4 ± 4.4 compared with 44.3 ± 3.5 µmol/L). In the dose-response study, the maximum increase in plasma vitamin C occurred three hours post dose in both men and women. Vitamin C concentrations remained significantly higher on days 7 and 14 than at baseline. Baseline concentrations of 8-epi-prostaglandin F2a (8-epi-PGF2a) were significantly higher ($P = 0.03$) among men than among women (249.6 ± 25.4 compared with 177.7 ± 6.2 pg/mL) but decreased significantly ($P = 0.04$) by day 14 of the intervention. A significant inverse correlation was observed between vitamin C and 8-epi-PGF2a (r = -0.791, P = 0.0022). Among smokers, baseline vitamin C was lower and 8-epi-PGF2a higher than among nonsmokers. This means that drinking orange juice (500 mL/d) increases plasma concentrations of vitamin C and reduces concentrations of 8-epi-PGF2a in humans. These effects were significantly more pronounced in smokers.

Many studies describe the protective role of vitamin C (ascorbic acid) against cancer development and in treatment of established cancer. The present study investigated whether ascorbic acid demonstrates a therapeutic benefit for prostate cancer. Androgen-independent (DU145) and androgen-dependent (LNCaP) human prostate cancer cell lines were both treated in vitro with vitamin C (0-10 mM). Cell counts, cell viability, and thymidine incorporation into DNA were determined. Treatment of DU145 and LNCaP cells with vitamin C resulted in a dose- and time-dependent decrease in cell viability and thymidine incorporation into DNA. Vitamin C induced these changes through the production of hydrogen peroxide; addition of catalase (100-300 units/ml), an enzyme that degrades hydrogen peroxide, inhibited the effects of ascorbic acid. Superoxide dismutase, an enzyme that dismutates superoxide and generates hydrogen peroxide, did not prevent decreases in cell number and DNA synthesis, suggesting further the involvement of hydrogen peroxide in vitamin C-induced changes. These results clearly indicate that reactive oxygen species (ROS) are involved in vitamin C-induced cell damage. However, that singlet oxygen scavengers, such as sodium azide and hydroquinone, and hydroxyl radical scavengers, such as D-mannitol and DL-a-tocopherol, did not counteract the effects of ascorbic acid on thymidine incorporation, which suggests that vitamin C-induced changes do not occur through the generation of these ROS. This means that vitamin C inhibits cell division and growth through the production of hydrogen peroxide, which damages the cells probably through an as-yet-unidentified free radical(s) generation/mechanism.

These results also suggest that ascorbic acid is a potent anticancer agent for prostate cancer cells (3).

The process of oxidation and reduction

Vitamin C is considered as a unique antioxidant in its type as it keeps the body in a chemical reduction condition. Some scientists see that vitamin C can work as an antioxidant that causes the cell's destruction. This hypothesis is correct, as the high doses of vitamin C are useful for our protection against cancer. The changes in the oxidation levels in the cells are considered as a main factor for the cancer evolution, and consequently the high levels of vitamin C prevent those evolutions and contain the canceration process; in addition, vitamin C operates as an antioxidant factor for the cancerous tissues and kills voluntarily the abnormal cells.

The oxidation and reduction operations in the cell have an important vital chemical particularity as the produced oxidation levels organize the genes and their programs. The cells use molecules like the upper hydrogen oxide as signals inside and between the cells, and the oxidation and reduction control some of the important factors in the cellular behavior that include the cell's development, reproduction, and death. This control is a phenomenon in all the multicells beings, and it is one of the important processes for controlling cancer. The important role here for vitamin C for the effective treatment of cancer originates from two dual factors—an antioxidant factor and an oxidation factor; and both the oxidation and reduction processes combine for controlling the cellular division and the cell's death. The high doses of vitamin C were found causing the necrosis of the cancerous cells for some patients.

Vitamin C and other antioxidants contain the cell's division and consequently prevent the cancer dangers by preserving the condition of oxidation and reduction in order to become antioxidant. There are some references that point to some genes that inhibit cancer as P53 that contains the cancer by the way of the antioxidant characteristic. On the contrary, the genes that activate the cancer, "the oncogenes," tend to increase the oxidation in the cell. There are other factors that cause cancer and activate it, like the X-rays and the ultraviolet rays that increase the oxidation and the reduction and cause independent and destructive fissures. The profusion in administrating vitamin C gives antioxidant free electrons and consequently contains the cancer evolution.

A nonpoisonous anticancer factor

An ideal treatment that activates the oxidation and reduction processes and depends on vitamin C for most of the patients who are not in the terminal condition is the following:

- three grams of vitamin C to be administrated five to six times daily in order that the daily dose reaches thirty grams. Here, it is recommended to use liposomes compounds of vitamin C.
- 200-500 grams of alpha-lebuic acid with each dose of vitamin C (five grams for the oral total dose of vitamin C).
- 4000 units of vitamin D daily.
- 800 micrograms of selenium daily.
- 400-2500 milligrams of magnesium daily (in the form of magnesium citrate).
- A diet very low in carbohydrates and very low in calories.
- A large quantity of fresh vegetables.

The cure of a cancer sickness case

The following sickness case was under the supervision of Dr. Andrew Saul in the United States of America. He was treating a sick man afflicted with cancer with high doses of vitamin C. The sick man named "Jo" was suffering from a lung cancer, and he was vomiting blood continuously. Dr. Saul talked to him in his bedroom, as he was too weak to go to Dr. Saul's clinic. The patient's condition was very critical; he could not walk, and he's enduring severe pains to the extent that he was not able to lie down in his bed, and he spent the whole night on a chair. The patient had no desire for eating, but he had a desire to live and wanted to try vitamin C if this will cure him. The time was in the autumn during the month of October, and it is not easy to deal with someone dying. As a consulting physician at Brigham Hospital in Boston, Dr. Saul suggested to the patient, Jo, to take vitamin C. The patient asked about the quantity, and the physician told him to take the largest possible quantity he can endure. Jo placed a large bottle of water next to him and a large jar of vitamin C. Within days, the coughing accompanied by blood stopped; and within a week, he recovered his appetite, and he could lie down in his bed. Gradually, his pains disappeared, and he managed to sleep with the line of patients being treated with vitamin C. After a week, patient Jo was able to walk around his home. His wife stated that his condition has improved due to vitamin C.

What is the quantity of Vitamin C Jo was taking?

The dose was about four grams every half hour when he is awake, night and day, and the total quantity per day was 100 grams. Jo did not suffer diarrhea. After sometime, it appeared that the vitamin C benefits for treating cancer can be increased by adding other food additives like the alpha-lipoic acid (thiotacid) and vitamin K3. Jo's condition improved, and he lived.

Cancer Research United Kingdom Molecular Oncology Laboratory, Weatherall Institute of Molecular Medicine reported that hypoxia-inducible factor (HIF) plays an important role in determining patterns of gene expression in cancer. HIF is downregulated in oxygenated cells by a series of Fe (II) and

2-oxoglutarate-dependent dioxygenases that hydroxylate specific residues in the regulatory HIF-a subunits. Because these enzymes require ascorbate for activity in vitro, they analyzed the effects of ascorbate on HIF in human cancer cell lines. Ascorbate at physiological concentrations (25 μM) strikingly suppressed HIF-1a protein levels and HIF transcriptional targets, particularly when the system was oncogenically activated in normoxic cells. Similar results were obtained with iron supplementation. These results indicate that both ascorbate and iron availability have major effects on HIF and imply that the system is commonly regulated by limiting hydroxylase activity under normoxic tissue culture conditions.

Digestive Diseases Research Centre reported that gastric juice vitamin C may be protective against gastric carcinogenesis, but concentrations are significantly reduced by Helicobacter pylori infection. The gastric cancer cell lines and various H pylori strains were treated with L-ascorbic acid for up to seventy-two hours. Cell viability and protein and DNA synthesis were determined. Flow cytometry was used for assessment of H pylori adherence, cell cycle distribution, and apoptosis. H pylori growth and its haemagglutination activity were determined using viability count and microtitration assay. The results showed that vitamin C induced a significant dose-dependent growth inhibition of gastric AGS and MKN45 cells, but this effect was significantly reduced at levels similar to those in gastric juice of H pylori-infected patients (<50 μM). Although vitamin C had no obvious effect on H pylori growth, haemagglutination activity or adherence ability to gastric AGS cells, as compared with untreated controls, significantly enhanced H pylori-associated apoptosis and induced cell cycle arrest in these cells. This means that vitamin C may inhibit gastric cancer cell growth and alter H pylori induced cell cycle events at concentrations comparable with those in gastric juice but has no effect on H pylori growth or pathogenicity. However, the inhibitory effect on gastric cancer cells was lost at vitamin C concentrations found in patients with H pylori infection.

References

1. **McCormick** B. "More on facing the reality of our aging population with breast **cancer**." *Oncology* (Williston Park). 26(9), (September 2012): 804, 806.

2. Edsall JT. "**Linus pauling** and vitamin C." *Science*. 178(4062), (November 17, 1972): 696.

3. Gröber U. "[**Vitamin C** in complementary oncology—update 2009]." *Med Monatsschr Pharm*. 32(7), (July 2009): 263-7. Review.

4. Flashman E, Davies SL, Yeoh KK, Schofield CJ. "Investigating the dependence of the hypoxia-inducible factor hydroxylases (factor inhibiting **HIF** and prolyl hydroxylase domain 2) on **ascorbate** and other reducing agents." *Biochem J*. 427(1), (March 15, 2010):135-42.

Part Two: Cancer Treatment by Food Medicine

Chapter Four: Nutrition against Cancer

Chapter Five: Therapy by Bees' Honey

Part Two

Cancer Treatment
by Food Medicine

Chapter Four
Nutrition against Cancer

Dr. Abdelfattah M. Badawi and Dr. Manal M. Khowdiary

Food Activation Power

ACTIVATION MEANS $1 + 1 = 3$ or 500, which is a very big value than 2; activation tells us that the joint efforts and effects of some factors result in an outcome greater than the expected. Do not depend on a magical prescription for a food substance to overcome your cancer . . . there is no such substance. Your body needs about fifty essential food substances in addition to one hundred food element with big value, which do not exist but in an integrated food supported with the perfect food elements.

Food activation means that when perfect food elements gathered together at the proper time in correct percentages, the body becomes an effective tool in fighting the disease.

Cancer Hunger

Cancer dines on sugar . . . You can slow down cancer growth by decreasing the quantity of fuel available for cancer cells. Higher and progressive glucose levels cause various diseases including cancer, diabetes, heart disease, higher pressure, and microbe diseases (1). Attempting to overcome cancer by eating food that increases glucose level is absolutely similar to attempting fire extinguishing at a forest where somebody is throwing benzene over the forest's trees.

Stop eating carbohydrates . . . Eat the kinds of food that contain fewer percentages of carbohydrates including fruits . . . Start a gymnastic program to burn blood glucose to reasonable levels.

Make fish and varied vegetables the main types of your food; have few quantities of fresh fruits in your food, knowing that it raises the blood glucose percentages. Have cinnamon because it helps in balancing the blood glucose; also, have food supplements such as vines and manganese.

Avoid malnutrition

Cancer is a disease that causes national loss, where over 40% of cancer patients die because of malnutrition, not cancer. Cancer secretes substances causing inappetence and in the meantime increases body needs of calories, thus resulting in cancer patient's loss of weight. You cannot fight agreement disease that threatens your life while suffering from malnutrition; you are in need of all food substances necessary to support your immune system which is your army in killing cancer cells. Also, remember that proteins are the backbone of the immunity system.

Though the radioactive and chemical therapies can kill cancer cells, they may generate multiple toxics against body cells. A cancer patient who has good food can protect the healthy cells against the toxic effects of radioactive and chemical therapies; thus he can make the cancer cells be affected with the chemical therapy.

Good nutrition can make radioactive and chemical therapies more selective in killing cancer cells and less destructive of natural cells (2-5).

Charge your immunity system

Your immune system is composed of twenty trillion cells, comprising security forces and sweeper forces of body wastes. It is in charge of killing any harmful cell including cancer, bacteria, and viruses. If you are suffering from cancer, it means that there is a defect in your immune system, which usually results from anxiety, toxics, and malnutrition (6).

Have good food and specific food supplements, lessen your anxiety levels, and use your imagination to imagine the immunity cells when they devour cancer cells. This is an effective experimented way. Remove toxic from your body, since toxics stand against the ability of your immune system to break the cancer cells up (7).

Body cells are divided billion times daily, resulting in composition of faulty cells; such faulty cells are divided into cancer cells, which can be identified by your immune system as cells having defect in their structure, and it devours them. The adult man passes six tours of cancer throughout his life. Life of 42% of humans ends at the cancer hospitals while 58% of people have a strong immune system that protects man from faulty cells. Therefore, make your immune system work and overcome your cancer upon appearance. Food products having the ability to activate the immune system including Lactoferrin, especially whey, aloes extraction, mushroom extraction (Mabtacky), beasts cells walls (1,3-beta-glucan), phytic acid, and Essiac Tea.

Healing power of integrated food

Throughout thirty years, scientists in USA have spent over forty-five billion dollars in their fight against cancer. However, nature has its healing powers since thousands of years (8,9). All of us have cancer all over the time, but the magic components of integrated food system are assisting the body to overcome cancer. Where ellagic acid existing in berry causes cancer cells to commit suicide, lycopene substance existing in tomatoes helps in restraining cancer growth, genistein substance in soybean, and glutathione substance in green leaves of vegetables, and S-Allyl cysteine substance in garlic . . . and many other substances acting as modern fighters of cancer in the twenty-first century.

All these anticancer miraculous substances stand in a waiting market:

- Have your food adjacent to its natural sources as possible.
- Have green vegetables as possible.

Nutritious appetite food

Pressure cookers, microwaves, and roasters are all marvelous methods for preparing appetite food. Some foods are nutritious if eaten raw such as many types of vegetables and most types of fruits (electric mixer is being used here in preparing nonappetite food and mixes them to compose a good appetite drink).

Try having two eggs and a half cup of cantaloupe juice in the breakfast meal, in lunch try a piece of grilled reconnoiterers with a sandwich of spinach, onion, and raw rice (brown) with a variety of colored vegetables added to Italian sauce, and the dessert with a half cup of strawberry. In dinner, you can have a piece of grilled fish with lemon, grilled potato, fresh tomato slices, and onion adding to Italian sauce and the dessert with a half cup of berry. All these are types of appetite food, and there are various meals in the same way.

Herbal medicine

For thousands of years, many herbs have been used in overcoming cancer; however, nothing of them is certainly the medicine of all cancers (10). There are many nontoxic herbs that motivate the immune system and have the ability to remove toxics. If you want to use essential herbs for cancer therapy, you shall start with fresh garlic as a seasonal food or to have garlic tablets.

There are many herbs that deserve attention such as astragalus, echinacea, goldenseal, glycyrrhiza, ginseng, ginkgo, and ginger, which have a golden value that help in curing you from cancer. Deal with an expert in herbal therapy to guide and assist you.

Useful fats

Many harmful fats have killed millions of Americans throughout the past fifty years; however, there are many new useful fats that have emerged such as, fish oil, primula oil, flaxseed oil (hot oil), and whale liver oil; all of these are helping in overcoming cancer (11-12). Simply start with a few capsules of fish oil on a daily basis; whale liver oil is more preferred since it contains vitamin A and vitamin D. You can prepare delicious food of Italian sauce using hot oil, olive oil, water, and vinegar.

Healthy fats in your food produce prostaglandin substances that serve in crumpling cancer; these useful fats work on the cellular lining membranes and decreases blood glucose via improving insulin performance. Healthy fats cause immunity cells to identify and destroy cancer cells.

References

1. Vin-Raviv N, Barchana M, Linn S, Keinan-Boker L. "Severe caloric restriction in young women during World War II and subsequent breast **cancer** risk." *Int. J. Clin. Pract.* 66(10), (October 2012): 948-58.

2. Aaldriks AA, Giltay EJ, le Cessie S, van der Geest LG, Portielje JE, Tanis BC, Nortier JW, Maartense E. "Prognostic value of geriatric assessment in older **patients** with advanced

breast **cancer** receiving chemotherapy." *Breast.* February 13, 2013.

3. Kim WS, Kim JW, Ahn CW, Choi SH. "Resolution of type 2 diabetes after gastrectomy for gastric **cancer** with long limb Roux-en Y reconstruction: a prospective pilot study." *J. Korean Surg. Soc.* 84(2), (February 2013): 88-93.

4. McGreevy J, Orrevall Y, Belqaid K, Bernhardson BM. "Reflections on the process of translation and cultural adaptation of an instrument to investigate taste and smell changes in adults with **cancer**." *Scand. J. Caring Sci.* February 6, 2013.

5. Montgomery K, Belongia M, Haddigan Mulberry M, Schulta C, Phillips S, Simpson PM, Nugent ML. "Perceptions of Nutrition Support in Pediatric Oncology **Patients** and Parents." *J. Pediatr. Oncol. Nurs.* February 4, 2013.

6. Sheth CH, Sharp S, Walters ER. "Enteral feeding in head and neck **cancer patients** at a UK **cancer** centre." *J. Hum. Nutr. Diet.* February 5, 2013.

7. Kirkwood JM, Butterfield LH, Tarhini AA, Zarour H, Kalinski P, Ferrone S. "Immunotherapy of **cancer** in 2012." *CA Cancer J. Clin.* 62(5), (September-October 2012): 309-35.

8. Ferruzzi MG, Peterson DG, Singh RP, Schwartz SJ, Freedman MR. "Nutritional translation blended with **food** science: 21st century applications." *Adv. Nutr.* 3(6), (November 1, 2012): 813-9.

9. Al-Naggar RA, Bobryshev YV, Abdulghani MA, Rammohan S, Al-Jashamy K. "Knowledge and perceptions of **cancer** and

cancer prevention among Malaysian traditional healers: a qualitative study." *Asian Pac. J. Cancer Prev.* 13(8), (2012): 3841-50.

10. Jia L, Jin H, Zhou J, Chen L, Lu Y, Ming Y, Yu Y. "A potential anti-tumor **herbal medicine**, Corilagin, inhibits ovarian **cancer** cell growth through blocking the TGF-beta signaling pathways." *BMC Complement Altern Med.* 13(1), (February 15, 2013): 33.

11. Busnena BA, Foudah AI, Melancon T, El Sayed KA. "Olive secoiridoids and semisynthetic bioisostere analogues for the control of metastatic breast **cancer**." *Bioorg Med Chem.* January 9, 2013. doi:pii: S0968-0896(13)00027-8. 10.1016/j.

12. de Miranda Torrinhas RS, Santana R, Garcia T, Cury-Boaventura MF, Sales MM, Curi R, Waitzberg DL. "Parenteral fish **oil** as a pharmacological agent to modulate post-operative immune response: A randomized, double-blind, and controlled clinical trial in patients with gastrointestinal **cancer**." *Clin. Nutr.* December 22, 2012. doi:pii: S0261-5614(12)00279-8.

Chapter Five
Therapy by Bees' Honey

Dr. Abdelfattah M. Badawi and Dr. Manal M Khowdiary

Acording to the Holy Book of Koran, the verse reads, **"In honey you find the cure."** Which proves the importance of honey, which is considered as a food full of vitality as mentioned previously, and it has its high importance in producing energy inside the body. People who account for honey in their daily food increase by all means their body and mind capabilities; sick people who need to reinforce their body are advised to add a spoon of honey to their breakfast.

Honey is a perfect food in case of weakness and indigestion, in case of convalescence after chirurgical operations, in severe sicknesses and poisoning, in duodenum, intestine, and children illnesses.

It is well known that honey has specification against putridity or infection. They are sufficient to influence on harmful germs inside the intestine. So as if the person substitutes meat and milk with honey for a long period of time, the group of harmful germs inside the intestines will decrease with a high percentage.

That is why it is advised in all cases of typhoid, ulcers, duodenum, and colon inflammation that the chosen food is based principally on honey.

Generally, the medical researchers have proved that bees' honey has a large effect on the digestive system and especially the stomach ulcer and the duodenum ulcer; it has been proven that by using 20 ml as a syrup three times a day daily before the meals will tend to cure the ulcer completely. As well as the irritation of the digestive system is cured by using honey. Some researchers have carried out works on some kind of bacteria which ulcerate on some wounds and resulted that honey kills those bacteria and helps in curing ulcerate wounds and also the permanent skin ulcers.

Bees' honey has the ability to help the aminic acid (methonin) to renew some parts of the liver deteriorated by the accumulation of some poisons. Honey prevents the accumulation of some fats resulting from the absorption of alcohols. It is well known that accumulation of fats in the liver weakens its functions and diminishes its work in sucking and breaking a lot of medicines and poison inside the body; that is why honey helps the liver in achieving its functions in a full picture and prevents it from some diseases like fibrosis and greasing.

Also, bees' honey influences fatness; researchers concluded that taking it with proteins lead to losing weight in overweight patients, in a better way and better results than that of medicines blocking appetite.

Honey kills germs

Bees' honey contains different minerals and vitamins needed by the body, and each component from the honey plays an important role for the human being's health protection. Honey has the ability to absorb humidity from any body bonded to it, even if it is a mineral or a hard stone. From life requirement is the humidity to stay in a living picture, and it includes also bacteria, and that by withdrawing the humidity needed for its life.

The bacteriologist who doubts in the ability of honey to kill bacteria has to test that and will discover for his surprise that when you put bacteria in bees' honey, it will die. The typhoid fever bacteria die during forty-eight hours. The germs which cause pneumonia die after four days while dysentery germs die during ten hours.

Honey as a sedative

Honey has a sedative effect on nerves, and if taken regularly, it improves the neurotic person; and for this purpose, it is advised to take a small spoon of honey six times a day.

The calming effect of honey has a value to those who suffer from insomnia as honey helps for a calm sleep. It is preferable to take honey in a hot drink before sleeping. That is why a small spoon or two of honey is added to a cup of hot milk (it has been noticed that the useful properties of milk are killed by boiling), or a large spoon of honey is added to a similar quantity of apple vinegar in a half cup of warm water, or honey is taken in warm water only. All of those drinks are tasty, and the best is the mixture of honey and vinegar.

Honey and vinegar

The mixture of honey and vinegar is described in the popular medicine in the United States of America and England to treat headache, high blood pressure, high-fatigue cases, sore throat, indigestion, and rheumatic pains.

Dr. Gavis from USA has registered cases cured as sinusitis and sensitivity by using the natural honey extracted directly from the beehive without any artificial treatment (some factories or persons boil the honey to facilitate bottling in recipients, but this boiling operation destroys most of the killing components inside the honey).

Honey and digestion

Fructose sugar found inside honey is of one unity composition and is easy for digestion and helps people suffering from indigestion. The normal sugar is called sucrose and is of two units composition and is transferred to one unity composition (glucose or fructose) when it reaches the intestines due to enzymes. This operation is carried out by the bee's saliva glands.

When you eat honey, it is absorbed easily and quickly without irritation to the membranes covering the digestive system; that is why we find that bees' honey helps to fulfill the normal operation of the digestive system. In addition, it works as a natural laxative.

A person having constipation can be treated by taking honey in a regular way in addition to fruits and fresh vegetables. Sometimes a mixture of bees' honey and molasses with equal quantities is prescribed as a natural laxative for treating constipation.

Honey and a weak constitution

Honey is a cure for a lot of illnesses or diseases, especially a weak constitution. Many different nations discovered the utilities of honey in treating many diseases. If you are suffering from any sickness and not responding to medical treatments, you have to try the honey.

It has been found that cough can be treated by using honey, and here are some experienced prescriptions.

Pneumonia cough

A mixture of equal quantities of honey and fresh lemon juice is used; also a mixture of honey and olive oil and fresh lemon juice is prescribed several times a day.

Permanent cough

A mixture of equal quantities of honey and flaxseed oil and vinegar is used, and the quantity is a small spoon for three or four times daily.

Influenza—responds to the treatment with a mixture of honey and vinegar plus large quantities of vitamin C.

Sore throat

Treated with a gurgle composed of one liter of water in which 125 grams of honey is diluted plus 25 grams of (قبش); this gurgle helps to treat the mouth ulcers.

It is possible to diminish the sore throat by using a mixture of two teaspoons of honey and a similar quantity of glycerin and a teaspoon of lemon juice and a little bit of ginger.

Honey helps also in treating the stomach ulcer and the colon inflammation. People working in beehives are the healthiest ones; they do not suffer absolutely from any kidney diseases, and they have a smooth skin and also a good vision, and they are not vulnerable to cancer or poliomyelitis.

Physicians have discovered that you cannot neglect the utility of honey for the heart. Dr. Thomas issued in an article in the scientific magazine *The Lancet* that honey has an impressive effect on weak hearts where it becomes more active in its motion and helps people with heart diseases to overcome their weaknesses. The heart is a muscle like any other muscle in the body, which becomes more active with honey and provides the muscle in fatigue with the necessary energy for its activity.

Honey, lemon, and tea are described for the treatment of kidney for skin diseases and influenza. The inflation of fingers due to cold weather is treated using a teaspoon composed of honey, glycerin, the white part of an egg, and some flour powder; this paste is spread over inflated fingers and covered with a bandage.

As a general fortifying, a drink composed of equal parts of honey, cod liver oil, and fresh lemon juice is advised. This composition is taken three times a day.

Honey as treatment of burns and wounds

In case of burns, honey can be used as it isolates the burned skin from air and reduces pain and prevents skin peeling. It also helps for healing the burned skin rapidly.

Honey has the ability to stop the blood hemorrhage as it works to speed the blood coagulation. Many ulcers and wounds are healed by using honey.

Bruises can be treated rapidly with a mixture composed of equal percentages of honey and glycerin, and this mixture is advised to be used to treat dryness of face and skin.

In the fourth century before Christ, the Greek doctor Abukrat mentioned the utility of honey saying, "It cures sores, ulcers, and relives lip sores and treats the spots on face."

Honey and children

All children like honey; that is why it must exist in their daily nutrition. Breast-feeding is the natural food for all babies. Moms who cannot, for a certain reason, afford to feed their children must provide honey in their daily child nutrition and add a teaspoon or two spoons of honey for every eight ounces (ةيقوا) of food. If the child has constipation, an extra spoon of honey is added (the quantity of honey is diminished by half a spoon if the child has a diarrhea). Children who have honey in their food are rarely suffering of indigestion.

A child's uncontrolled pee in bed is a great problem for many mothers; this act is treated by honey with its ability to absorb and keep the humidity. If the child gets a teaspoon of honey before going to bed, it will calm him and will reduce wetting his bed in the morning.

A child must not get sugar in any phase of his age phases because sugar reduces the child's growth and exposes him to many diseases during his growth phases. Dr. Seil Harris commented about that by saying, "The child who introduces sucrose in his nutrition is facing the colon irritation and the infectious diseases, and he becomes pale in color and weak in constitution." Children increasing sugar are facing the following symptoms: acidity, headache, continuous motion, tooth decay, constipation, diarrhea, rheumatism, eczema, enlargement of throat glands, and asthma; you can prevent all those harmful effects by exchanging them with honey.

Honey as an old treatment

Honey has been known as a food loved by people from old history, and it has been used as a treatment from long ages; honey is propagated in past times in China, India, the Arab countries, and Europe. And its use is registered in ancient books.

History has registered the use of dead bees for treating the eye sicknesses. It has been mentioned in some old books that pure honey containing dead bees, if a drop is put in the eyes, will make it pure. It is also true for the honey mixed with bees' heads.

In old descriptions for treating baldness, it has been said that an ointment of the head's bald part with honey mixed with bees' heads helps the growth of hairs another time.

Honey and beauty products

Honey and beeswax are essential for manufacturing skin creams, lipsticks, and skin lotions. It is possible to do a lotion for treating hand's dryness at home by mixing the white part of an egg with a spoon of glycerin and one ounce of bees' honey and a little bit of flour. This ointment is kept in the refrigerator for using it when necessary.

Cream of beeswax can be prepared easily as follows:

Fifty grams of white beeswax in 140 milliliter of paraffin oil in a temperature of fifty degrees and heated in 120 milliliters of distilled water and adding four grams of borax. This mixture is added to the melting wax in the paraffin oil, and the blending is continuous till the mixture turns to a heavy constitute. A perfume can be added during blending.

A paste for the face skin can be produced by mixing the honey with half a cup of flour to do a homogeneous paste (rose water is added to lighten the paste constitution); the face is cleaned completely, and the honey paste is spread over it and be left for a period of thirty minutes, and then the paste is removed with a piece of cloth wet by hot water. Using this honey paste twice weekly will keep the skin face smooth, fresh, and pure.

Pollination grains and the royal food

Honey is not the only product of bees that is useful to man. The honey cake and bee wax and pollination grains and royal jelly are all bees' products with many utilities.

The bees collect in their trip the pollination grains and the flowers scent ريحق and bring them to the hive to use it as food. Pollination grains are very rich in protein, and without the grains, the bees cannot make their function peacefully. Bees cannot live without the pollination grains. Man can use pollination grains in his meal and is available abroad as honey cake or mixed with honey; it produces activity and vitality in man and is described in convalescence periods after sickness.

It has been found that pollination grains cure from some health symptoms as brain hemorrhage, anemia, weakness, intestine and colon irritation, poisoning, constipation, insomnia, loss of appetite, depression. But the royal jelly is honey in a jelly form eaten by the bee queen. If eaten by a human being, he will feel activity and vitality. The royal food has a big value as treatment for heart weakness.

Honey cakes

Chewing the honey cakes has a big value as treatment from sensitivity sickness as the straw fever hurting the respiratory system with asthma; honey cakes also cure the nose sensitivity and the sinusitis pockets. The effect of honey cakes is very rapid, because if chewed, the blocked nose returns to normal in a very short time.

Dr. Garvis has mentioned in his book about popular medicine that children using honey cakes in their food till reaching sixteen years are rarely hurt by cold or sensitivity; chewing the honey cakes generates immunity in the respiratory system, which continues for four years. One can benefit from honey in advanced age if the human being is chewing the honey cakes in a regular way.

People who are suffering from sensitivity sicknesses may chew the honey cakes daily for a period of one month before the spring season where the sensitivity crisis increases. This treatment will either prevent sensitivity completely or reduce its sharpness. During the sensitivity crisis, the patient must chew the honey wax daily. It is advised to chew the honey wax daily regularly after that to prevent the sensitivity crisis in the following year.

The propitious quantity of honey wax is a teaspoon in one time or to fill the mouth with honey wax if you are chewing the gum and to continue chewing for fifteen minutes and throwing the remaining outside the mouth.

Bee poison

Even the bee bite has medical utilities. There is a belief within farmers in Europe that the bee bite cures the rheumatism. But it is not proved surely till now. It is dangerous to try to cure from the bee bite if the patient has sensitivity to bee poison; there is one person for every thousand persons who has sensitivity against bee poison. Every bite makes the sensitivity worse and may lead to death. Any person having sensitivity against bee poison may be treated on the spot.

We can discover the sensitivity of bee poison by testing the blood, and the patient's treatment depends on taking a dose of reduced poison vaccine gradually till the body acquires immunity against the bee poison.

Bee is a good food

In some places, bees do not live in zones of the north of the United States of America, having very cold winters where complete colonies of bees die and hives are kept till the next spring.

The colony contains around five pounds of bee's buds; (تاقري النحل) these blights have a nutrition benefit as they are rich in protein and vitamins A and D. These buds are made ready for marketing. There is a product called "small bees," which are bee's buds that are fried and kept in a sauce inside special boxes which are exported from Japan to the United States of America.

At Alberta University in Canada, some researches and experiences are carried out to conserve and prepare large quantities of bee's buds which are collected from the forests of Canada; those researches comprise the methods of refrigeration, drying, smoking, frying, and cooking. The people having tasted it prefer bee's buds roasted, and they taste like chestnut and sunflower seeds and roasted rice.

Honey against cancer

Studies have proven that bee's honey has a countereffect against cancerous cells in urinary bladder in testing tubes. Also on test mice by injecting bee's honey of 6-12 % or directly through mouth (1).

There are many experiences which showed large curing properties of bee's honey against bacteria, fungus, and irritation; results have shown effectiveness against stomach ulcer, burns, and cancer, as by injection of mouse having cancer (Ehrlich ascites) with doses of bee's honey of (10, 100, or 1000 milligram/1000 gram of mouth weight) day after day for four weeks had an effect against cancer because of an increase in the number of cells of bone's spinal cords and blood white cells (Macrophages) (2).

Another international research has been issued recently proving the effectiveness of bee's honey, rich in different phenolates, in its countereffect against different types of cancer including colon, stomach, uterus, brain, and leukemia cancer. This research has been carried by a team of Indian scientists and has been diffused internationally (3).

Another research issued in 2010 proved the effectiveness of bee's honey, rich in different phenolates, toward the cancerous cells Ehrlich ascites and the hard cancers in animals (4).

References

1. **Swellam T**, Miyanaga N, Onozawa M, Hattori K, Kawai K, Shimazui T, Akaza H. "Antineoplastic activity of honey in an experimental bladder cancer implantation model: in vivo and in vitro studies." *Int. J. Urol.* 10(4), (April 2003): 213-9.

2. **Attia WY**, Gabry MS, El-Shaikh KA, Othman GA. "The anti-tumor effect of bee honey in Ehrlich ascite tumor model of mice is coincided with stimulation of the immune cells." *Egypt J. Immunol.* 15(2), (2008): 169-83.

3. **Jaganathan SK**, Mandal M. "Antiproliferative effects of honey and of its polyphenols: A Review." *J Biomed Biotechnol.* 2009;2009: 830616.

4. **Jaganathan SK**, Mondhe D, Wani ZA, Pal HC, Mandal M. "Effect of honey and eugenol on Ehrlich ascites and solid carcinoma." *J. Biomed Biotechnol.* 2010;2010: 989163.

Part Three: Water against Cancer

Chapter Six: Alkaline Water Treatment and Elevating Body Alkalinity

Chapter Seven: Oxygen Water against Cancer

Part Three

Water against Cancer

Dr. Abdelfattah M. Badawi and Dr. Manal M Khowdiary

TWO-THIRDS OF OUR body is composed of water, and the water is considered as the greatest material on the earth's surface that provides the life liquid in our bodies; in addition, water acts like a bath that washes all the cells in the body. Most people do not obtain their sufficiency of water, yet they drink polluted water. The polluted water is considered as a time bomb as the result of the pollution from rivers, lakes, and oceans with huge quantities of poisons; and the scientists consider that the water sources' pollution is one of the reasons of cancer affliction.

Buy for yourself a good water filter and install it on a water faucet in the kitchen. This water filter should be provided with two layers of carbon in addition to the reverse osmosis pressure membranes (RO); and if you don't have a filter, use the mineral water bottles, but here you should be cautious because some of the mineral water bottles in the markets are filled with faucet's water.

Drink large quantities of water in order to lighten the urine to become clear in color and not malodorous. The chronic dryness leads to the crispation of skin, a weakness in the concentration, constipation, and repeating diseases afflictions, which may lead to the appearance of cancer. Drink large quantities of clean water.

Most materials dilute in water; water is available in any place, at a cheap price, and not poisonous if it is clean. Water absorbs a large quantity of heat. Water stores energy. Water moves from the liquid condition to gaseous or solid state and has advantages in all three states.

More than 70% of the body contains water, and water has the following characteristics:

- Water is the highest spreading among the compounds (it contains 90% hydrogen and approximately 10% oxygen).
- Water can be shaped, as it can touch every part of the human body inside and outside.
- Water absorbs and lets out a large quantity of heat.
- The healthy benefits include:
  — It was proven scientifically that drinking water prevents cold affliction.
  — It improves fertility and treats chronic tiredness and activates the immunity system.
  — It improves the heart and blood circulation functions.

The water bath

It was proven by clinical experiments that taking a regular cold bath every day for two minutes has the following benefits:

1. It increases the body's immunity against cold affliction.
2. It increases the body's hormones production and helps in men's and women's fertility.
3. It renovates the energy for the persons who suffer from the symptoms of chronic tiredness.

4. It improves blood circulation and also the enzymes level in the body.

5. It decreases the affliction of heart attacks as it helps to get rid of the clots in the blood arteries.

6. It increases the level of the white blood corpuscles, and consequently it helps in activating the immunity system against diseases.

7. It improves the nails' solidity and the hair's growth.

Water is your friend. You should drink large quantities of clean water.

The treatment by water free of deuterium

The water molecule is composed of one oxygen atom and two hydrogen atoms; and the normal water contains 150 molecules in a million of deuterium, the radiating hydrogen isotope, and it is acceptable for the people. The scientists noticed that decreasing the deuterium level has an effect on the cancerous cells, as it leads to destroying them (1-2).

In some clinical studies in Budapest, Hungary, the effect of the treatment with water free from the deuterium isotope was shown. The study was conducted on seventy patients who were treated with the traditional anticancer medicines in addition to the water free of deuterium. The statistics showed positive benefits for the group drinking water free of deuterium in comparison with group drinking normal water containing deuterium in addition to the disappearance of the side effects of the chemical therapy.

This discovery opened new horizons for the cancer treatment, and the precaution from it after the completion of a comprehensive study on 1,200 patients with cancer presented positive results regarding the treatment and precaution against most types of cancer.

Due to the continuous pollution of the drinking water, the radiating deuterium ratio reached one deuterium atom for 6,400 hydrogen atoms. Some distinguished scientists announced that the deuterium accumulation in the human body causes the speeding of aging and diseases affliction; as with the increase of the deuterium average an imbalance in the reactions inside the body cells happens, and consequently it hastens the division operation, and the possibilities of the cancer appearance increase.

The disposal of deuterium water

The deuterium water molecule D_2O freezes at 3.82°C, while the normal water molecule freezes at 0°C. There is a Russian company that managed to dispose of the deuterium water by freezing it, as the frozen water that contains most of the heavy deuterium water is disposed of.

A glass container of one gallon capacity is filled with filtered water until it reaches two-thirds of the container capacity. The container is placed in the refrigerator with the necessity of having a small opening in the container cover to enable the water, when it dilates at the freezing point, to leak out through this opening.

The necessary time for forming a shuck of ice over the water in the container is supervised, knowing that the ice will be formed on the container walls. The not frozen light water that contains water free of deuterium is separated through the container opening in another container, and the formed ice that contains heavy water rich in harmful deuterium is disposed of. Afterward the light water free of deuterium is placed in the freezer until it freezes completely. The container is taken out and placed in the sun until the frozen water melts and drinking bottles are filled with it. This water is a cure and a treatment for several diseases, and it is a precaution against cancer and antiaging.

References

1. Wang H, Liu C, Fang W, Yang H.Nan Fang Yi Ke Da Xue Xue Bao. "[Research progress of the inhibitory effect of **deuterium**-depleted **water** on cancers]. 32(10), (October 2012): 1454-6. Chinese.

2. Wang H, Zhu B, Liu C, Fang W, Yang H.Nan Fang Yi Ke Da Xue Xue Bao. "[**Deuterium**-depleted **water** selectively inhibits nasopharyngeal carcinoma cell proliferation in vitro]." 32(10), (October 2012): 1394-9. Chinese.

Chapter Six

Alkaline Water Treatment and Elevating Body Alkalinity

Dr. Abdelfattah M. Badawi and Dr. Manal M Khowdiary

Acidic Remnants

MOST HUMAN DISEASES arise from a mere single source, namely, acidic remnants. The point is how to recognize whether your body organs are overly acidic.

It man in need of blood, urine and saliva tests 7; nowadays there are no accurate tests to reveal the body's acidity as the popular testing means only revealing the present acidic remnants in the body fluids (blood, lymph fluids, urine, mucous, and saliva). And these tests fail to provide reliable results regarding the actual quantity of acidic remnants within the body organs, as the body fluids are in a perpetual flow within the tissues in a feat to dispel the excess acidic remnants.

And although it is possible to assess the body fluids as to their alkalinity or acidity, it is, however, impossible to evaluate the body's condition (skin organs, glands, muscles, ligaments, veins, and arteries) based on blood, urine, and saliva tests.

Unfortunately, the acidic remnants are duly expelled and become reabsorbed via the colon onto the liver and therefrom to the circulatory system where they are precipitated in the tissues; such precipitations designate illness or affect health; it is therefore necessary to identify the acidic remnants in the body in view of having the body liberated therefrom.

It is thereby possible to attain a distinctive health and an energy and power that enable man to enjoy life.

Body Alkalinity and Acidity

The chemical principle underlying the reactions leading to alkalinity and acidity in the body are by no means vague processes. And a simple understanding of such processes forms a reliable means capable of overcoming pertinent problems or rectifying their divergence.

In this section, questions concerning the disorder in the state of equilibrium between alkalinity and acidity as a potential cause of many scientific problems we confront are given herein:

1) How are alkalinity, acidity, and pH value defined?
2) Why are information concerning reactions leading to alkalinity and acidity in the human body considered of utmost importance, and how do such reactions influence man's well-being?
3) What are the materials and conditions pursuant to alkalinity and acidity reactions in the body, and the reason therefor?
4) What is it that impedes the suitable alkalinity and acidity equilibrium in the body?
5) What are parameters of daily nutrition and lifestyle that can be followed to ensure the suitable alkalinity/acidity ratio in the body for the highest health fitness?

The Alkaline Diet

The ideal food to eat are fresh or raw food as they contain enzymes that are readably digestible. When such enzymes are deficient, the body pansies them liver. The stored quantities of these enzymes in our bodies is, however, limited. Therefore, upon consuming our cooked meals, we should supplement it with digestive enzymes.

It is also ideal that we eat 75% of our food fresh and 25% cooked. Start with food of which 60% is fresh and 40% cooked. Continue following this 60%:40% ratio till you are sure that your body has become oriented to consuming excessive fresh foods.

Then gradually transfer to the 75%:25% ratio.

The following diet is a well diet and is well known to produce body mucous (enhances its aspiration), but try to reduce or to avoid such diet.

1) All chemically processed foods or those conserved by satirizing or saluting.
2) Meats.
3) Dairy products.
4) Wheat.
5) Eggs (except raw eggs).

Why Reduce Meats?

Because they contain hormones and free radicals and a large quantity of neurotic predicators which cause it to centralize in the brain and affect the glands (1).

Why Reduce Dairy Products?

Because milk, particularly the pasteurized and processed brands, leads to a rise in the risks of an increase in the body acidity in case it is not a direct output from the farm cattle to the babies nourishment. Pasteurized meat maximizes the outcome of those risks.

Why Reduce Eggs?

Eggs are risk developers too (generating acidity). The exception thereto, and which is considered a diet of high value for the brain, is to eat the egg yolk (the alkaline product). Lecithin and cholesterol are found in the yolk in balanced amounts and does not constitute a risk to the health as long as it is not hard-boiled or and not mixed with the egg whites.

Overboiling the eggs destroys the lattices and develops acidic products. It is therefore recommended to eat the egg yolk in the raw form or in the slightly boiled state. Also avoid eating more than six eggs per week, and be sure that they are of an organic origin.

Why Reduce Wheat?

The fluting found in wheat forms a glue in the intestine and leads to its blockage. Eat in your meal, alternatively, rice, corn, or soya beans, which is the alkaline acidic joint diet.

It is recommended to eat melon (alkalinity developer) separately, or at least twenty minutes before any meal. Melon is digested quickly in the intestines when mixed with other food ingredients; in the intestines, such mixture penetrates promptly followed by its fermentation.

Vegetables and Fruits

Don't mix fruits and vegetables in a single meal. Fresh fruits are digested quickly in the fine intestine (75-90 minutes) while some vegetables last three hours to be digested. Don't mix fruits with starches.

Water: The Healing Elixir or the Lethal Poison

Distilled water and alkaline waters are nowadays considered the mostly acquired necessity.

We, however, strongly object the idea of drinking distilled water because

1. distilled water withdraws the valuable metals from your body,
2. it withdraws minerals from salt, and
3. it deprives you from important minerals which you need from spring waters.

Everyone possesses different levels of acidic remnants in his body organs. And distilled water merely enhances fully negative ionic reactions in the body organs. And negative ions are alkaline.

And forms of water contain various amounts of positive ions (acidity constituters), except for water that has been reconverted into alkaline water. And the acidic remnants found in the body tissues, which lead to the extermination of the cells, are positively charged. And distilled water induces an array of negative charges, which attract the positively charged acidic remnants, driving them toward the body's disposal conduits.

Over several years, poisonous remnants have gushed into the soil. And there are exit evidences advocating the seeping of detergents, formed chemicals, and even radioactive materials into water sources. Also, factories all over the country dispose their industrial wastewaters which exceed the permissible levels of pollution.

Experts, in this respect, recommend not to drink city town water. It is quite sufficient to note the amounts of residues that precipitate when we fill a glass with tap water.

Disinfecting chlorine in this water dissociates to be converted into chloroform; and the aluminum constituted in alum, and which exceeds the levels permissible in potable water, is associated with many diseases in accordance to relevant reports published by trusted scientists.

The minerals contained in all sorts of water nowadays are not of biological constipation, and the body consequently doesn't benefit from them, thus being converted into acid-forming remnants in the tissues. Mineral water includes eighty-four identified minerals of natural sources and are moreover free from any hazardous bacteria.

And the acceptable alternative of distilled water is reversed osmosis water. But the relevant filters become contaminated with time, and untreated water constitutes a hazard on the body's alkaline reserves and disturbs the appropriate alkaline equilibrium.

And the most recent discovery regarding potable water nowadays is the alkaline water constituted electronically.

Electronically constituted water is produced by means of a special unit fixed to the tap, and this system produces alkaline potable water. It, moreover, has further advantages, in that it reduces water coagulation, i.e., the water molecules are reconstituted into simple lighter molecules which are more readily absorbed in the body. Consequently, you don't merely obtain a more alkaline source bat; there are also modifications in the aqua vibrations which are considered of paramount benefit. It would be possible to use the acidic outlet in this device as an epidermis antiseptic. In this regard, several health spas worldwide have been provided with such units.

Positive clinical results have been realized for many of those who have used the units electronically constituting alkaline water, knowing that such technology has conferred hygienic benefits upon many who have used it over a number of years. Moreover, electronically produced alkaline water is accompanied with complementary vibrations inexistent in distilled water.

The alternative choice would be to drink distilled water on condition of adding alkaline minerals, as adding ten drops of mineral metals in eight ounces of distilled water results in an approximate 0.8 pH value.

Life Ambiguity and Aging

Analogous nucleic acid nuclei (DNA) reproduce the various organs in the human body. In other words, the analogous nucleic acid cells reproduce hair on your skull, while they reproduce fingernails on your fingers.

Knowing that each of your body cells comprises the same nucleic acid found in an original individual cell. And all your cells are provided with information sufficient to build up everything in your body (bones, skin, teeth, eyes, heart, blood, etc.)

Malignant carcinogenic cells may be termed "cells that have lost their intellect" as they promote the reproduction of things beyond their concern. And this principle raises many intriguing questions:

- How do such cells lose their intellect?
- Can such intellect be maintained within the cells?
- How can the body cells be accessed?

The Commencement of Aging

Buildup and demolishing processes on-going in the body, and the oxidation (combustion) of food in view of obtaining occupational energy, generates waste residues which the body endeavors to dispose. The question at this point is how can we completely dispose such wastes?

In fact, the wastes that cannot be completely disposed become stored in our bodies in a certain place. Knowing that the aging process, which will commence as of the dawn our lives, is but the accumulation of these wastes which haven't been disposed.

The body endeavors to eliminate the poisons accumulated within it and disposes them.

Eternity

Since the old eras, people have been in search of eternity. And history tells us that every civilization and every human kind has been in search of the spring of youth which would provide them a more lengthy life. From the theoretical point of view, we can be considered to be eternal. For the ovum and the spermatozome combine to form novel cells and a new life—in other words, immortal viral, all part of which survive to reproduce a new life. And in accordance to the science of new life functions, viral cells don't show aging symptoms and possess within them the power of life from one generation to the next. We further possess other types of cells considered the body's normal. When these cells grow, they become converted into specialized tissues. Nerves, muscles, cartilages, cords . . . skin, bones, and fatty tissues. These tissues grow further in the form of specialized organs. Unfortunately, these tissues and organs are all oriented to reach an advanced aging age and wither. What causes the withering of these all?

The Aging Process

The answer here is quite simple. Cells dissociate due to the accumulation of waste materials. Can you imagine a house in which 99.9% of the waste it produces every day is not being allowed to be eliminated? After a few months, the house shall be infested with obnoxious smells. We now grasp that the aging process and the dissociation of cells is a result of the accumulation of wastes in the body. We now have to find a safe means that enables the body to daily dispose these wastes. So if we can now succeed to somehow withdraw the old wastes which our bodies have stored since a few years. We shall vanquish aging and become ever more youthful.

Abating the Aging Condition

We by no means mean here to return age backward. Neither do we imply here as well to eliminate the wrinkles so that you might have a youthful appearance whilst your innermost self is on its way toward aging. Abating aging implies reduction of the wastes for a fifty-year-old body to that levels of a forty-year-old body or maybe younger. So that if the wastes haven't caused an irreversible destruction of the body tissues and organs, it would thenceforth be possible to restore its functional vitality

Water and Life

Water is known to maintain life in all forms, including man's life. And in this regards, water may be considered the most obscure material upon this planet. And many scientists are still on their way in discovering amazing facts about water. More than 70% of our body's weight is made up of water; this may be interpreted by saying that a person weighing 120 lbs encloses ten gallons of water so that you are none other than a package of water maintained within your skin through which it flows.

To perceive water and to drink the proper kind thereof will grant us both health and youth.

Properties of Water

Water is a powerful solvent and thus holds much unseen materials (minerals, oxygen, foodstuffs, wastes, pollutants). Within the human body, we find blood (90% water) flowing throughout the body to distribute food and oxygen while collecting the wastes and carbon dioxide. And every sort of materials within the depths of our bodies has been introduced via water and can be driven out also via water. Water is of lighter density in the solid state than in the liquid state. Thus ice floats on water. And water not only maintains life but also protects.

Water Composition

The water molecule (40) is composed of two hydrogen a (H_2) and one oxygen atom (O); the two hydrogen atoms are not linked to the oxygen atom at an 180° angle but at a 104.5° angle in the liquid state, and at a 109.5° angle in the ice-solid state; thenceforth, ice is less in density.

Such angles develop an electrical polarity in water. And the oxygen radical is considered more on the positive polarity than oxygen. Consequently, water molecules form compounds of changing on hexagonal to pentagonal configurations, alternating a very short time (10 to 11 parts of a second) recurrently).

Water Is Alive

Yes, indeed water is inherently alive, without there being anything within it alive. Knowing that the percentage of the hexagonally configured water molecules change by heat.

In pure water, there are three to four hexagonal water molecules at 10°C. At 0°C, the 10%, percentage ratio is reaching 100% at 40°C, knowing that the flakes are of hexagonal configuration.

Water Is a Living Organism

The scientist Dr. Shan registered in the science and technology center in the city of Seoul in South Korea an important fact that the protein molecule is surrounded by some 70,000 water molecules, such molecules constituting at least three different layers of different configuration. He termed those three layers "X, Y, Z."

The water layer adjacent to the protein layer was termed Z, where the outermost large layer was termed layer X, and lying between them was a large Y layer. The water layer Z is considered to be linked to the protein molecule by an ionic bond, resembling solidified water, only that it doesn't freeze other than at very low temperature.

The large outermost layer X is far from the protein layer's zone of influence and freezes at 0°C.

Whereas the next layer Y, freezes at a temperature of -10°C. Studying this layer is of extreme importance, as it enables us to understand the hygienic actives and enzymes in the living organs. For example, the intermediate layer Y surrounded by a molecule of the amino aniline acid and is 62% hexagonally configured, 24% of pentagon configuration, and 14% other configurations.

Here we can say that hexagonally configured water may be considered the water of affinity to living organisms. This explains why water outlets from ice suit the growth of planktons and green algae. This is because water produced from ice contains large amount of hexagonal configuration; such results are not readily observed, but have been disclosed and simulated by means of computer-aided programs.

And Dr. Shan explains that the Y water layer, which surrounds a malignant carcinogenic cell, is not comprising many configurations; and he interprets in one of his studies that ionized calcium institutes a hexagonal configuration for the water entering it.

Other Water Properties

Scientists have found that water has a memory to a certain extent. And when water is exposed to a magnetic or an electrical field or to quantum energy, it acquires properties of surface for balance and configurational activities as compared to other liquid substance. This phenomenon enables our bodies to resist various heat fluctuations.

In addition to that, we note another property of water that is ionization. Ionization takes place when an atom or molecule loses electrons or gains them from another atom. And not withstanding an absence of any mineral in the water, one in a ten million molecules of the water molecules is in a state of ionization. And when water molecule ionizes, the H_2O molecule dissuades into two molecules (a positive H^+ ion and a negative hydroxyl OH^- ion).

These ions in turn ionize the minerals in the water, whence an active chemical reaction is set up and whereas water causes ionization; our body in absence of water doesn't host any chemical reaction which means death.

Acidic and Alkaline Water

There are sometimes some positive hydrogen ions H^+ exceeding the negative hydrogen ions OH^-. Here water grade is termed acidic. Conversely, water which contains more negative OH^- hydroxyl ions than positive H^+ hydrogen ions is termed alkaline water.

When the relevant numbers are equal, the water is termed neutral. There is important hypothesis with respect to the number of positive H^+ hydrogen ions and the negative OH^- ions.

When water is neutral at its normal ambient temperature, then the ratio positive H^+ hydrogen ions in relation to the total number of water molecules is 1:10.

Assuming that the total number of water molecules to be one unit, then the total number of positive H^+ ions in this neutral water is 1×10^{-7} units. Shortly, we can say that the hydrogen concentration in the water is 0.7.

Upon adding acidic materials such as sulphur or chlorine to such water, positive H^+ ions increase because hydrogen atoms donate electrons to the acidic metal. Hydrogen concentration of this water is 0.6. The positive hydrogen H^+ ions concentration is always measured in order to determine the acidity or alkalinity state of the water.

Alkaline water is distinguished by containing less positive H^+ ions than negative hydroxyl OH^- ions. Such water contains more oxygen atoms than half of the hydrogen atoms. Conversely, acidic water contains positive hydrogen H^+ ions more than negative hydroxyl OH^- atoms. Such water contains less oxygen atoms than half the hydrogen atoms.

Human blood's hydrogen concentration ranges between 7.3 and 7.45. This implying that blood of 7.45 hydrogen concentration contains 64.9% more oxygen than does blood of 7.3 hydrogen concentration. Hydrogen concentration values of 7.3 and 7.45 are similar, though there is a major difference in the quantity of excess oxygen as regards with this values.

Excess Oxygen in Alkaline Water

Identifying the hydrogen concentration values of various drinks, we can measure the positive hydrogen H^+ ions and the negative hydroxyl OH^- ions in a glass of water. The following table represents a comparison between the hydrogen concentration values and the percentage ratio of excess oxygen in ten ounces of various drinks.

Drink	Hydrogen Concentration	Percentage ratio of excess oxygen
All Cola drinks	2.50	-185.1×10^{20}
Carbon pitted drinks	2.20	-31.55×10^{20}
Filtered water (RO)	6.80	-0.005×10^{20}
Distilled water	7.00	Zero
Filtered tap water	8.40	-0.12×10^{20}
Alkaline water	10.00	-5.0×10^{20}

All types of carbonated drinks are highly acidic, especially cola drinks.

And in order to neutralize a glass of cola, twenty-two glasses of strong alkaline water are required.

Defense Devices

Tap waters in towns have different characteristics. And in order to eliminate the bacteria and microbes, chlorine is added to the water. Chlorine is considered a good antiseptic, but is harmful if swallowed in big quantities.

Moreover, chlorine combines with the hydrocarbons found in water to form carcinogenic chlorinated hydrocarbons. That being the most widespread pollution problem worldwide. The most effective filters for chlorine and chlorinated organic materials are the charcoal filters. As compacted charcoal filters and the granulated charcoal filters are the most widespread filters. But the major disadvantage of the latter granulated charcoal filters are that they rely on the surface adsorption of chlorine and the chlorinated hydrocarbons, knowing that are no mechanical constraints to any solid grains in the water.

Upon consumption of all the charcoal, the filter supplies unfiltered, whence operator is held to assess the chlorine in order to learn whether the filter is still functioning.

This type of filters is usually provided furnished with a silver coating to avoid the accumulation of bacteria in the filter. Whereas for compacted charcoal filters, these do not only allow the elimination of chlorine and chlorinated hydrocarbons, but harness of the water flow in order to trap heavy metal particles and bacteria.

The only drawback in these filters is that the water pressure drops with the continued use of the filters.

The Super Defensive Killing

Man can wear a steel armor to an extent rendering him unable to move, which enables his enemy to kill him. This is called the super defensive killing.

In an attempt to obtain pure water, some people employ a purification device and a reversed osmosis filter. This type of filter affects everything from the water. Unfortunately, this water is considered unhealthy. It is lethal water in which fish can't survive. And upon extended use of this water, it extracts the valuable body minerals such as potassium, magnesium, sodium, and calcium. Besides that this water doesn't include excess oxygen.

The Aggression System

The old-age problem results from the acid wastes in our bodies. The target should be to help our bodies to get rid of the acid surplus wastes. As those wastes are carried by the blood and disposes of them in a liquid form; therefore drinking quantities of healthy water type is very important for our health. And the best type of water is alkaline water free from acidity, which is the water that equilibrates the harmful acid wastes and expels them without taking out from it the valuable alkaline metals as the potassium, magnesium, sodium, and calcium.

The necessary device for supplying the alkaline water free from acids is called the water ionizer. This device allows supplying the body with alkaline water that will reverse the old-age process and will prevent the affliction from many diseases.

The Cancer Cells Development

The German chemistry scientist Dr. Otto Warburg discovered the cause of the recurring of the cancer in 1923. He obtained the Nobel Prize in 1932. He indicated in his researches the "photosynthesis for the tumors." The main cause for the cancer is the oxygen substitution in the breathing chemistry for the normal cells by the sugar fermentations. The cancerous cells development is considered as a fermentation process that is created by the relative shortage of oxygen. It is not yet known the cause of the oxygen shortage in the human body.

The hydroxyl -OH supported by positive ionized alkaline metals. If you hold your breath, the oxygen stops and you die. Also, if your body acidity decreases to less than 7, the oxygen (O_2) stops and you also die. When the breathing stops, the oxygen (O_2) is consumed first, and death happens. This takes three minutes. The persons having high alkalinity, like children, live longer than three minutes.

By returning to the German and Japanese researchers, what happens in our bodies is the following: when the cells environment becomes very acid, this means that there is no sufficient oxygen for the adjacent cells. For those cells to live under those conditions, they supply some cells optionally with carbon dioxide and expel the oxygen (like the plants), and at that time a temporary destruction for those cells occurs and causes them to live deformed for a longer period, and this transforms to cancerous cells.

The Best Protection Methods against Cancer

To drink high-alkaline water helps a lot for preventing cancer. There is a no-return point. But as the healthy cells are alkaline, and the malignant cells are acid, therefore to drink alkaline water will not harm the healthy cells, while it destroys the malignant cells.

The body acidity starts in the blood that works on balancing the blood alkalinity in the limits of 7.2 to 7.45. The blood has an alkaline reserve of sodium bicarbonate for equalizing the acid compounds resulting from the cells as wastes resulting from the food photosynthesis process. When this reserve decreases, the acidity starts appearing and also the different diseases (1).

The Acidity and the High Blood Pressure

The Japanese scientist Dr. Koninaka, one of the pioneers of treatment by alkaline water in Japan, announced that the high blood pressure patients have an acidity case in the blood. He recorded many successful clinical cases by using the alkaline water for treating the high blood pressure.

The scientific interpretation for this is that the blood high alkalinity is accompanied by surplus oxygen, making the blood not exerting much effort. The other factor is that viscosity of the high alkalinity blood is usually low, making the heart not exerting much effort for pumping the blood. Another reason is that the calcium ions in the alkaline water may be diluting the sedimentations and the accumulated cholesterol on the arteries vessels, and consequently it increases the blood flow.

The physicians know very well that taking a deep breath several times before measuring the blood pressure makes the blood pressure reading low, and the interpretation of this is that the breathing increases the blood alkalinity momentarily and in the exhalation process for expelling the carbon dioxide, and in the inhaling process for inhaling more oxygen. The person suffering from his high blood pressure may decrease his high blood pressure in a few months by drinking alkaline water.

But if your blood pressure is always high, this is due to your narrow arteries (angiosclerosis), and the treatment by alkaline water will take longer time, and it may one year or more for diluting the sedimentations and the accumulated cholesterol on the arteries, but it will happen after some time.

The Diabetes

The Japanese scientist Kuwabasa treated successfully diabetic patients by using alkaline water. He recorded the case of a patient aged forty-nine years who was suffering from diabetes and having a treatment depending on insulin. And by using alkaline water, the sugar level after a month decreased to a tangible level after that this level was high reaching 300 milligrams.

The pancreas produces secretions distinguished by the highest level of acidity among the body liquids. This leads to that the blood is transformed into an acidity condition that harms the blood arteries and causing clogs as the result of an increase in the proteins causing the defect of the pancreas functions. The alkaline water helps for treating this case by supplying the pancreas with calcium in the form of ions and also by preventing the accumulation of the proteins sedimentation.

And with aging (which we know now as the accumulation of the acid wastes) the pancreas efficiency decreases, and it is clear that the acid wastes accumulate in men more than women, and consequently the men start building amino acids around the body waist.

It is known that the heredity plays a role in the person's ability for the accumulation of the acid wastes near the pancreas. And when reaching the age of forty years, the acid wastes accumulations will be sufficient for slowing the pancreas function, and this means that if you can prevent this accumulation the person will not be subject to diabetes, even if he reaches the age of eighty or ninety years.

The treatment by alkaline water does not apply to the adverse diabetes cases in which the pancreas is not functioning.

The Gout Disease and the Arthritis

Most of the gout cases forms are the result of the acid wastes accumulation in the joints, and the heavy weight persons have a higher pressure on their joints, resulting in the tearing of their ligatures; but in young ages, this does not appear. Nevertheless, the acid wastes accumulation are the ones that destroy the cartilages and inflame the joints, and for our bad luck we find that in the joints area, the blood cannot dispose of those wastes.

The gout results from the uric acid accumulation in the joints. It is a disease resulting from a malfunction in the food photosynthesis and is distinguished by uric acid surplus in the blood and sedimentations of uric acid in the tissues around the joints especially in the feet and hands and causes severe pains especially in the big toe. The sooner we accept the fact that those diseases are the result of superfluous acid wastes, the faster the treatment of such problems.

Nowadays, we find many advertisements for ointments that relieve the pains of the arthritis patients. Finally the physicians recommend the change of the type of diet, and is a step in the right direction, and drinking the alkaline water changes the acidity condition in a way in which the body confines those problems by itself.

Mrs. (Jenny) wrote from Florida saying that due to the water conditions nowadays, she and her husband, aged sixty-five and sixty-seven years were suffering from some health problems; so they installed the best water filter in the market since many years, but with no result. After they read about the water ionizer that produces alkaline water that removes poisons from the body organs, they installed this device six months ago.

Her husband was suffering from a high level of uric acid, and he was also diabetic, and this caused him to be afflicted with gout and arthritis. He was suffering from pains in his hands, fingers, knee, and all his joints; and the pains prevented him from playing golf and other activities. Now he is not suffering from any pains after drinking the alkaline water, and he stated that he couldn't live without it.

The Kidney Diseases

The more the body produces acid wastes, the kidneys become more overcharged, and they should dispose of those acids out of the blood. The rise of the uric acid and all the bladder diseases are all disease cases related to the acidity, and they can be improved by consuming alkaline water. This water helps in adjusting the osmotic pressure in the kidneys that form stones of phosphorus and uric, and usually they are united with calcium and magnesium ions. They are formed in the kidneys because of the acid environment.

Drinking a lot of alkaline water may form the kidney stones, but even after their formation this water will dilute them.

The Bones Fragility

The bone skeleton is considered as the "bank for the calcium element," and the body condition becomes acid; it compensates the calcium by recuperating it from the bones leaving them fragile and easy to break.

Many aged persons are prone to the transformation, and they look shorter as they become older, and this is due to the loss of calcium from the bone skeleton. The long-term use of alkaline water helps to prevent this destruction resulting from the modern diet. The ionization helps a lot for repairing this malfunction.

The Eyes Diseases

We do not consider the change of our eyesight with old age as a type of disease, and we accept this as an established fact. The question here is, "How and why this happens?"

With the accumulation of phosphorous salts and uric acid in our cells, this makes them lose more oxygen, and this causes an incomplete combustion of the sugar in the cells; and this causes its connection with protein molecules, and the result of this is that the cells and tissues become dry, hard, and not flexible.

The question here is, "Can we revert this process?" The answer here is that drinking alkaline water daily and cooking for several years will remove the old accumulated acid wastes from the cells and will improve the eyesight.

The Methods of Reverting Old Age

All the foods create wastes inside our cells and tissues after the food photosynthesis operation. Our style of life does not allow our body to dispose of those wastes completely. The accumulation of the wastes is the explanation of old age. Therefore reverting the old age is just the process of getting rid of the old accumulates wastes in our bodies. Those wastes are acid, and consequently our bodies are transformed into more acidity with the advancement of age. Reverting the old ages requires two separate processes—a chemical process and a physiological process.

The chemical process

It works on lowering the acidity in the body for enabling it to dispose of the acid wastes in the blood and cells safely and easily.

The physiological process

It is the disposal of the old wastes stores in the blood vessels so the body can get rid of them.

There are several methods for reverting the old age. Among the known ones is the alkaline diet (vegetarian diet and the macrobiotic diet). They are chemical diets. As for the physical exercises, they are considered as a physiological process that helps to dispose of the acid wastes in the body.

The Chemical Aggression

Due to the main problem being too much acidity, the solution is to pump alkaline metals in the body. Generally the vegetables and fruits are considered as alkaline foods in the body, while the grains and meats including poultry are foods forming acidity (2).

The Foods Forming Acidity

They include the foods causing acidity in the body according to their descending order in acidity: rice, egg white, brown rice, poultry, oysters, salmon, wheat flour, escalope, pork meat, beef meat, cheese, barley, shrimps, beans, bread, chicken soup, butter, asparagus.

From this classification, we see that the tuna and egg white are more acid at the ratio of two to four times than the beef meat. The beef meat has special enzymes required by our body that we cannot get from any other food.

The Foods Forming Alkalinity

They include (according to their descending order in alkalinity) ginger, green beans, spinach, soya beans, bananas, nuts, carrots, mushrooms, strawberries, potatoes, cauliflowers, radish, sweet potatoes, orange juice, apples, pears, grapefruit juice, melons, coffee, onions, tea, human milk, cow milk, tofu.

The Balanced Diet

Some people follow a vegetarian diet or macrobiotic diet, and this for the purpose of decreasing the body acidity, and this is not easy; therefore it is recommended to follow an acceptable and balanced diet. All the foods have different tastes, and each one has unique elements inside them; therefore it is difficult to stay away from them, and the deprivation from a specific food may create a deficiency in its important elements. As we do not know exactly what the body absorbs, the sacrifice will be to eat all kinds of food and leave to your body intelligence to determine what he wants.

Drinking Alkaline Water

The experts recommend that we do not use a specific food for removing the acid wastes, but instead of this to use alkaline water to sweep away those wastes. Enjoy various kinds of food but the right type of water in order to dispose of all the wastes. And as the wastes we are trying to dispose of are acids, therefore the right type of water is the alkaline water (3).

A glass of alkaline water of a hydrogen concentration of 10 contains 2,110 negative hydroxyl ions (-OH), and each one of them is united with positive ionized metals, like the calcium, magnesium, sodium, and potassium. And as the alkaline water contains calcium more than any other water, therefore it is assumed that it is rich in calcium ions amounting to 33.2 milligrams in one glass.

Drinking five glasses daily of alkaline water will make the body acidity to decrease and enable the body to dispose of all the acid wastes that are accumulated daily. To drink ionized alkaline water is much better than taking alkaline metal pills as the calcium pills.

The Making of Alkaline Water

The alkaline water is made by a water ionizer that electrically separates the filtered water into alkaline water and acid water. The water ionizer started to be discovered at the beginning of year 1950, and the experiments were conducted on animals and plants. In year 1954 the faculties of agriculture in Japan started a comprehensive development on the effects of ionized water, and especially the acid water on plants.

The experiments on the human body lasted a long time because of some difficulties in the researches' continuity. In spite of this and with continuous and long-term experiments by the Japanese scientists, the valuable data was gathered, proving that the alkaline water produced by water ionizer is not harmful and was able to treat many old-age diseases.

In year 1958, the first water ionizers at a commercial level appeared in Japan, but they were not available as large units in the hospitals. In the year 1960, a team of physicians in Japan established medical specialized institutes, and they held annual conventions for registering their discoveries. And finally in January

15, 1966, the Japanese Ministry of Health approved the water as a medical device that helps improving the human being's health.

In the year 1970, the Japanese water ionizers were presented to Korea, and the South Korean government approved them as medical devices. And in year 1985, the Korean water ionizers were presented for home use to the United States. They were tested on April 15, 1986, and it was proven that the alkaline water resulting from the water ionizer is free of any harm according to the American Federal Developments Agency.

The Ionization

The water ionizer contains two compartments with positive and negative electrodes. The negative electrode pulls to its compartment the positive metals that are the alkaline metals, while the positive electrode pulls to another compartment the negative metals that are the acid metals. We find that water going to the water ionizer contains positive and negative metals mixed together, but after the ionization operation, we find that one compartment has only alkaline metals, and the other compartment contains only acid metals. Both compartments are separated by a special membrane with very fine holes that do not allow the passage of the water molecules, but allow the passage the passage of the nonorganic ionized metals. The ionization operation occurs when the water goes through the water ionizer. The water ionizer does not add any chemicals or metals to the water; it only ionizes the present metals in the water and separates them to the alkaline side and the acid side (4). The alkaline water seems turbid, but it becomes transparent within seconds and resembles the spring waters rushing from the mountains.

The alkaline water is considered good for cooking and making tea and coffee, and any alkaline water used in cooking rice equalized the phosphorous with calcium before eating it, and therefore it prevents the formation of the phosphoric acid that may result from the rice afterward in the human body.

Many antiaging scientists say that they are searching for the "youth spring," but no one of them searches in the drinking water, and the worst is that they drink carbonized drinks that hasten aging.

The Alkaline Water Is Not a Medicine

We have to remember that the alkaline water is not a medicine nor a food, and what is recommended is to drink alkaline water so it flushes the acid wastes which are the principal reason for the aged person's diseases. A caution is to be taken from the carbonized drinks, especially the cola because it is acid and causes many diseases with the age advancement.

References

1. **Song Ruixia, Xing Shuxia, Bai Xuetao. "Safety assessment and effect of new-type drinking water on immunity in mice."** *Journal Hygiene Research*. **4-2004.**

2. **Griffiths, J.R. "Are cancer cells acidic?"** *Br. J. Cancer* **(1991), 64, 425-427.**

3. **Li Yepeng, Han Chunhui, Li Yanjun, Li Yuwei, et al. "Impact of extra waters on immunosystem in mice."** *Journal Hygiene Research*, **4-2004.**

4. **Fu Rufang et al. "Effects of mineral water on the immunological function of mice."** *Journal of Radiological Health*. **3-1998.**

Chapter Seven
Oxygen Water against Cancer

Dr. Abdelfattah M. Badawi and Dr. Manal M. Khowdiary

THE TREATMENT BY hyperbaric oxygen is very expensive, as the costs of a unit reaches 100,000 dollars, while the treatment with oxygen water costs just a few dollars. It was used for treating emphysema, AIDS, and also cancer.

The use of the oxygen water by injecting it in the vein palliates the sensitivity diseases, the influenza diseases, and the critical viral afflictions, as this leads to the oxidation of all the strange materials in the blood.

The cancerous cells, the bacteria, and the undesired materials in the blood can be destroyed by the treatment with oxygen water. The oxygen water has a harmful destructive effect on the cancer cells, and the cancer treatment is considered as its greatest useful method for the treatment by oxygen water.

You came to life crying, but is it obligatory that you leave this life also crying? Many physicians think that the use of oxygen water is for just the external use or for dying the hair to a blond color.

The scientist Walter Grotz is among the first group of men who tried the oral treatment with oxygen water (1). His rheumatism condition improved within sixteen days by using the oxygen water, and the treatment did not cost more than six dollars.

In 1940 in India, the physicians Andergat Singh and Mangaldas Shah in Bombay used oxygen water in the vein. The use of oxygen water in the treatment dates back to 1916, as it was first mentioned in the medical magazine *The Lancet*, as a scientist named Feinstein mentioned using successfully the oxygen water for treating dogs in France, and they did not have any side effects. And in 1916, the two scientists, Turncliff and Estebing, used the pure oxygen in the vein for the first time on a human being, and they stated the following conclusion: "the use of oxygen water in the vein if applied cautiously will be available for the treating physicians, and it will give important positive medical results."

The Indian physician Singh treated the killer diphtheria at that time by using the oxygen water as a spray in the nose, and Dr. Singh noticed that the dogs could live for sixteen minutes with treatment by oxygen water in the vein without any air in the lungs. He tried applying this treatment with sick persons about to die from pneumonia at that time. Out of six cases one survived.

A German physician names Regelsberger recorded about the use of oxygen water in the vein for treating the high blood pressure, and he recorded a decrease in the blood viscosity and a decrease in the blood pressure.

In 1930, Dr. Oliver and Dr. Cantap published in *The Lancet* magazine the use of oxygen water in severe cases of killing pneumonia for soldiers with hopeless expectations for living. 50% of them were saved, and thirteen out of twenty-five survived, and all of them were supposed to die without oxygen water.

The method for using the oxygen water as a treatment is summarized in that the toxins resulting from the bacteria or viruses are oxidized by the oxygen.

The oxygen water is not poisonous, and it is the basis for life. There is a critical case that will result in death if an intensive treatment with antibiotics and hyperbaric oxygen is not used. This case is the gangrene that occurs as a result of the contamination of wounds and surgical operations, as the bacteria generates a gas that invades the tissues, so the tissues inflame enormously as the result of the gas formation and a malodorous odor results from the afflicted tissues, and if not treated the patient dies within forty-eight hours.

Like the cancerous cells, the bacteria that cause gangrene proliferate without oxygen, and therefore the ideal treatment will be intensive doses of antibiotics with hyperbaric oxygen.

In New Delhi in India, two Indian physicians inflicted dogs with the gas gangrene in their legs. One group of dogs was treated with oxygen water in the vein at the place of the affliction, and the other group did not receive this treatment. For this group their tissues and muscles decayed and they die from septicemia, while for the group that was treated with oxygen water ten dogs survived and only two dogs died.

How the Oxygen Water Affects

The oxygen water that is scientifically called hydrogen peroxide is a transparent liquid, nonodorous, and dilutes in water in all concentrations, and its diluted solution is with a ratio of 3%, and the oxygen water is used in the following:

1. As a whitening agent.
2. As an antiseptic and sterilizing material.
3. As an oxidizing agent.
4. As an oxidizing agent in the small jet engines.

The oxygen water decomposes at the rate of 1% monthly; also it is unstable, and even when it is heated it decomposes slowly, and at the decomposition reactions that increase in the presence of metals and glass it may explode. The cold makes the decomposition slower, and because of this it can be preserved and stored at below zero degree. The oxygen water is found in scarce quantities in the nature, and generally in rains and snows (2).

The first studies on the injection with oxygen water were expecting that the age will be less than one second, but the recent studies by MacNaghten found that it is half the age to become ¾ second to two seconds according to the rate of its mixing with the blood.

The oxygen water reacts with the catalase enzyme in the plasma and the white blood globules, and then it penetrates the cellular tissue to the red blood globules and reacts with the catalase enzyme in them, as additional oxygen is freed afterward.

The killing biological activity of the oxygen water is due to the interferon. The natural killing cells in the human body produce this interferon that is prepared by the oxygen water.

A comparative study was achieved between administrating oxygen water under pressure to the patient, and giving him oxygen water in the vein for studying the level of the oxygen ratio in the tissues. It was discovered that it was the same ratio in both cases, and the importance of this is due to that treatment operation by oxygen under pressure is very costly, and it has some dangers, and in general not available. On the other side, the vein injection with oxygen water is available, costs less, safer, and more effective.

After two hours of the vein injection with oxygen water, we find that 2-10% of the blood components decrease, like the sodium, potassium, chlorides, and phosphorous, after twenty-four hours those components return to their original condition.

The water oxygen is a strong oxidizing agent, and it oxides the both poisonous and nonpoisonous materials. The scientist Farr describes the biological effect of the vein injection with oxygen water as an oxidative detoxification. Among the benefits of the oxidizing operations is that they include the fat materials oxidizing on the wall or the blood arteries walls to reflect the arteries hardening operation. The peroxide is considered as the natural cells ammunition in the person for killing the bacteria inside the body.

The oxygen water as a mouthwash kills the bacteria and delays the gingivitis and decreases the formation of lime. The studies proved that the oxygen water affects the syphilis, fungi, viruses, and even the parasites.

The Middlesex Faculty of Medicine in London performed experiments on the oxygen water for treating the malaria, and it proved its effectiveness.

The oxygen water molecules are amazing ones. The cells that attack the contagion in the human body produce oxygen water as a first defense line against every type of fine particles that invade the human body as the parasites, fungi, and bacteria. There is no chemical compound that can reach the oxygen water effectiveness in its importance for the life. The oxygen water enters in all the vital operations for life and is present in the synthesis operations for the proteins, carbohydrates, and fats, and also the synthesis of vitamins and metals, in addition to the immunity in the human body, and anything related to the life functions; and all this needs oxygen water molecules.

There are approximately 6,100 examples in the scientific references since 1920 until now about the practical applications for the oxygen water, and in the mysterious operation that was not totally determined, the devouring blood white globules secretes oxygen water, and therefore it devours the adverse bacteria. The oxygen water works also like the insulin by transporting the sugar through the body.

The oxygen water is important and even more important that the thyroid gland as for generating heat in the human body. In the presence of the auxiliary enzyme Q10, the heat is generated between the cells, so it warms the cells and it is a basic operation for life.

The water oxygen is essential for fabricating the materials that are similar to the hormones, which are called the prostaglandin. Also vitamin C operates to produce oxygen water to help the production of prostaglandin, and this explains the effective role of vitamin C for treating the reactions of inflammation, and its protective ole against the contagion resulting from producing the oxygen water, which in its turn produces prostaglandin.

The Researches Proved the Oxygen Water Effectiveness

In 1960, a team of physicians from the Medical Center at Taylor University performed a series of studies on the oxygen water on animals and human beings. One of their studies concentrated on treating the cancer of the body tissues, and they are more sensitive to the radiation treatment if the oxygen concentration in those tissues was a high concentration. It was presumed that the oxygen water in the vein injection moves to the cancerous regions and makes them more sensitive to the radiation. The cancerous cells do not like the oxygen, and therefore there are two forces operating against the cancer, the oxygen and the radiation. The medical team recorded a positive effect from this marriage that is called a radiation treatment that affects with low doses.

The oxygen water decomposes very quickly as it enters the blood circuit, and the oxygen is freed in less than a second (1/10 of a second), and consequently the blood becomes sufficient with oxygen and this is called (hyperoxia). In this operation, the ratio of the freed oxygen is four times the oxygen resulting from the treatment by oxygen under high pressure.

The scientist Finney and his colleagues proved that the oxygen water injected in the arteries of a sick man suffering from arteriosclerosis helps a lot in removing the fats from the arteries walls and avoid for them the painful, dangerous, and costly bypass operation.

The victims of heart attacks usually die within hours of the attack in which the heart beats quicken and become in a turmoil condition as a result of responding to the lack of oxygen in the heart, which is called (hypoxia). Calming the heart and using electroshocks, and administrating usually do the treatment of such cases, and administrating the drug lidocaine in the vein. It appeared that the oxygen water has a stimulant effect on the heart muscle as it makes it to beat with more vitality and efficiency (inotropic effect). The heart that collapses in pumping blood in the blood circuit usually is saved by oxygen water. The lack of oxygen in the heart muscle (myoccirdial aseinia) usually improves by the oxygen water. The chaotic rhythm in the heart muscle that results in death was totally improved by using the oxygen water.

The experiments were executed on rabbits then on pigs, then on the human being. The first experiment was performed on a lady aged sixty years suffering from a collapse of the blood circuit for an unknown reason, and it resulted in unnatural heartbeats and a critical drop of the blood pressure. And within a minute of injecting the oxygen water in the vein, her heart recovered its normal beats and the blood pressure returned to the normal level.

In 1967, the medical team of Baylor Center faced the case of a patient aged sixty-five years suffering from a stroke as the result of the clogging of the main neck artery; the patient's condition was worsening with the normal treatment, and then she started being treated with oxygen water in the large artery of the neck (carotids) with the hope that the injected oxygen will succeed in reaching the deep fine arteries in the bones and muscles inside the neck vertebras. The patient was treated with approximately 100 oxygen water injections along twenty-eight days. Within a week, the patient's condition as of the movement coordination and the talking, and she managed to sit without a vertigo happening, in addition to the improvement of her blood globules count.

There is an experiment conducted by Dr. Finney and his assistants, and this by making the rabbits to inhale oxygen water mixed with a salt solution. The result was the doubling of the oxygen ratio in the blood compared to using the compressed oxygen.

Chemically, the oxygen water is decomposed into water and oxygen according to the formula:

$$H_3O_2 \longrightarrow O_2 + H_2O$$

The Oxygen Water and Cancer

The cancer treatment by radiation is a two edged weapon. In many cases, the cancerous block shrinks, but at the same time it lowers the patient's immunity system—meaning that the treatment succeeds in making the cancerous cells to shrink, but at the same time it lowers the patient's life expectancy.

There is a direct relation between the oxygen quantity in the cancerous block and the treatment effect by radiation. The more the oxygen increases, the more the radiation kills the cancerous cells.

The Baylor Medical Team injected the artery leading to the cancerous tumor with oxygen water, and therefore it becomes more able to be destroyed by radiation. One hundred and ninety patients were studied by using the injection with oxygen water in the artery leading to the cancerous tumor. The experiments lasted six years, and the results were amazing.

There was a sick man aged eighty-eight years who had a cancerous tumor in the mucous membrane of the right cheek (as a result of smoking), and he was treated by leaking the oxygen water in the neck artery leading to this cancerous tumor. The patient lived and became free from cancer for six years afterward. The hypothetical age for this patient without treatment was twelve to eighteen months.

And there was the case of a young man aged twenty-nine years suffering from a cancerous block (fungating) under his jaw. He was treated with the same method by leaking the oxygen water to the cancerous block, and accompanied by a radiation treatment. The report results in 1967 were that the patient lived and became free of cancer.

Can the oxygen water be taken orally?

Dr. Edward Defuria, a great scientist, is the first one to suggest taking the oxygen water orally; and the composition he suggested is still considered as a standard one. Many people recommend taking the oxygen water orally, and it is benefiting orally, but there are cautions or using it this way. The vitamin S, the iron, and the fats in the stomach change the oxygen water to independent fissures of (superoxides) making them to cause harms to the membrane lining the stomach. The experiments conducted on mice with low concentrations of oxygen water showed the dangers of taking the oxygen water orally, as it caused corrosion to the membrane lining the stomach.

The oxygen water is cheap and the pharmaceutical companies can register it, but it will threaten the antibiotics industry (as it has an effect as an effective antibiotic). And it will also threaten the industry of the heart arteries transplant industry (bypass) (as it cleans the hardened arteries), and it will also threaten the surgery industry and the chemotherapy treatment of cancer (with the exception of the treatment by radiation and oxygen water that reduces quickly the cancerous tumors with the lowest poisonous dose of radiation).

I have friends who thank for using the oxygen water orally, and friends who complain from using the oxygen water orally. All what I am asking for is that you decide by yourself.

If taking the oxygen water orally affects the stomach, may be the dose is high or incrementing, and you have to decide the suitable dose and timings for you. The practitioners using the oxygen orally attest that they did not face any problems.

My conclusion about taking the oxygen water orally is that it is not dangerous as long as the recommended dosage does not exceed ten points of oxygen water with 3% concentration, three times daily.

Dr. Charles Farr sees not to take oxygen water orally when there is any food in the stomach. He recommends taking it on an empty stomach. Sometimes there are reactions from it with the bacteria and the formation of poisons resulting from their decomposition, which is known as the (Herxheimer) reaction, and this ends after some treatments.

The skin inflammation is considered as a good relation that may frustrate the patient, and the patient may suffer from unnatural tiredness, insomnia, nausea, or diarrhea, and this differs from one case to another that they are being treated.

There is no general condition for the oxygen water reactions and any small expected reactions, and according to the doses and the number of times can be reduced, but the patient should not stop, and the result is that the patient will be cured and in good health. Before you start consult a specialized physician, and this will not be easy even with the physicians using the oxygen water by injecting it in the vein, as they will not be enthusiastic for recommending to taking it orally.

Dr. Charles Farr Experiments

Dr. Charles Farr performed some experiments for proving the treatment effectiveness by the oxygen water in the vein and that is not wasted in the two lungs.

This physician proved that injecting the patient in the vein with oxygen water by using the most advanced scientific devices:

1. It increases the food synthesis rate.
2. The extension of the small arteries.
3. The oxygen that is decomposed from injecting the oxygen water stays on the blood circuit and is not wasted.

The patients subject to those experiments recorded a mental awareness, acute eyesight, and an increase in the shining of the external middle and a feeling of relaxation.

Dr. Charles Farr recorded an important improvement in many of the severe cases that included microbe afflictions, sensitivity, and influenza.

Presently, Dr. Charles's group and his assistants are performing the dual treatment for the oxygen water and the claw treatment by using EDTA. The two factors cannot be mixed due to the side reaction that results from mixing the oxygen water with other compounds. Dr. Charles invites the experienced physicians in the treatment with claw materials to participate in a national study by using this dual treatment, which is called (the C1111``lelox therapy). All the experts and physicians across the United States of America and several other countries established a volunteering organization (not aiming for profit) for supporting and encouraging advanced researches in this new field that was called (bio-oxidation), and this organization is called "The International Oxidative Medicine Association."

The Oxygen Water and the Immunity

Dr. Charles recorded a clinical remark which is that after the patients received several repeating treatments of vein injections with oxygen water their condition improved, the patients with sensitivity to pollens and foods, and also the improvement of the patients afflicted with pneumonia, asthma, and chronic sinusitis.

Dr. Charles recorded a decrease in the immunity cells that are transformed to cells at the rate of 55% during twenty-four hours after the vein injection. The immunity cells are the one producing the antibodies. The process with which the vein injection with oxygen water for alleviating the sensitivity diseases is unknown.

The random choice of the sensitivity patients for this study at Dr. Charles's clinic was performed. The IGA, IGM, IGE were performed before and after the vein injection with oxygen water, and it was proved the existence of a clinical improvement for those patients as the result of the immunity globulins.

Afterward Dr. Charles studied the antibodies for Epstein virus (EBV) and the Candida fungus that were measured before and after the treatment by vein injection of oxygen water. Usually the patients receive twenty sessions weekly as per the following: a weekly session for a period of ten weeks, five sessions for a month, then repeating a weekly session for ten weeks. The antibodies were measured before and after twenty treatment sessions, then after three months, then after six months—a clinical improvement appeared accompanied by a decrease in the antibodies level for all the patients, and they were a group of patients of EBN virus (accompanied with a chronic tiredness).

A noticeable improvement in the energy and endurance appeared with a decrease of the complaints about tiredness. Also the group of patients with Candida fungus witnessed a clinical improvement accompanied by a decrease in the level of the antibodies to the Candida fungus after the treatment of vein injection with oxygen water.

In another study on the self-sensitive antibodies that cause the rheumatoid diseases of all types (arthritis, lupus, sekrodermia . . .), Dr. Charles found in all the studied cases that the antibodies do not appear after ten sessions or more of vein injection with oxygen water. This discovery confirms the principle of the vein treatment with oxygen water for lowering the B and T cells in the blood circuit, and the decrease of the globulins is accompanied by a clinical improvement for all the patients.

The oral treatment program with oxygen water of 25% concentration

The peroxides are supposed to be harmful to the human being as they form independent fissures and others, but now we hear that the oxygen water (hydrogen peroxide) has a benefit.

The oxidation treatment in which the oxygen is pushed in the blood under pressure lowers the patient's life in the poisoning cases by carbon monoxide or the poisoning by cyanide. The operation of using the oxygen under pressure in the blood is costly, and the cost of one unit of concentrated oxygen amounts to approximately 100,000 dollars, while the oxygen water costs just a few pounds.

The treatment by increasing the oxygen concentration in the blood is effective in the cases of cancer, emphysema, AIDS, hepatitis, and others.

The increase of the oxygen concentration in the blood treatment reduces quickly the sensitivity reactions, the influenza symptoms, the severe virus afflictions, and this oxidizing the harmful strange materials in the blood. The cancerous cells, the bacteria, and many of the harmful materials in the blood can be usually destroyed by the treatment with oxygen water. The oxygen water has a destroying effective effect on the tumors. And it was proved the cancer response to this treatment as the American physician William Campbell Scott stated:

- The following are the suggested doses for the treatment by oxygen water one hour before eating, or three hours after eating:

A large spoon of pure water is used with those doses, and when reaching large doses it is possible to use a greater quantity of water. When the patient feels nausea at any dose, he has to stay on this dose or return to the preceding dose.

First day	To use 9 drops	(3 drops three times daily)
Second day	To use 12 drops	(4 drops three times daily)
Third day	To use 15 drops	(5 drops three times daily)
Fourth day	To use 18 drops	(6 drops three times daily)
Fifth day	To use 21 drops	(7 drops three times daily)
Sixth day	To use 24 drops	(8 drops three times daily)
Seventh day	To use 27 drops	(9 drops three times daily)
Eighth day	To use 30 drops	(10 drops three times daily)
Ninth day	To use 36 drops	(12 drops three times daily)
Tenth day	To use 42 drops	(14 drops three times daily)

Eleventh day	To use 48 drops	(16 drops three times daily)
Twelfth day	To use 54 drops	(18 drops three times daily)
Thirteenth day	To use 60 drops	(20 drops three times daily)
Fourteenth day	To use 66 drops	(22 drops three times daily)
Fifteenth day	To use 72 drops	(24 drops three times daily)
Sixteenth day	To use 75 drops	(25 drops three times daily)

For severe cases:

To continue with the dose of twenty-five drops three times daily for a period of one to three weeks. Then gradually down to the twenty-five drops two times daily until the disease case improves, and the treatment lasts from one to six months.

For ordinary cases:

• The following can be applied:
Then twenty-five drops every two days four times daily
Then twenty-five drops every three days
Then twenty-five drops every four days
Afterward a preserving dose of 5-15 drops is taken weekly.

The Possible Side Reactions for the Oxygen Water

Nausea, insomnia, weakness, diarrhea, cold in the head, affliction in the ear, and this as the result of the body getting rid of the poisons; and this is a natural result as the body is cleaning itself after the bacteria's death and disposing of it through the skin, the lungs, the kidneys, and the bladder. We should remember that when the oxygen water touches the virus or the streptococcus bacteria, it generates free oxygen, and this may happen inside the stomach.

References

1. Altman, Nathaniel and Rochester, Vt. "The oxygen prescription: The miracle of oxidative therapies." Healing Arts Press, 2007.

2. Clarke, WB and Blackman, WW. "Hydrogen peroxide therapeutic use." United States: s.n., 1886.

www.ingramcontent.com/pod-product-compliance
Lightning Source LLC
Chambersburg PA
CBHW022013170526
45157CB00003B/1226